MEAL PREP COOKBOOK

Amazingly Easy, Delicious & Low-carb Recipes for Beginners

(Keto Meal Prep Recipes for Weight Loss, Fat Burning and Healthy Living)

Robert Elliott

Published by Alex Howard

© **Robert Elliott**

All Rights Reserved

Meal Prep Cookbook: Amazingly Easy, Delicious & Low-carb Recipes for Beginners (Keto Meal Prep Recipes for Weight Loss, Fat Burning and Healthy Living)

ISBN 978-1-990169-70-0

All rights reserved. No part of this guide may be reproduced in any form without permission in writing from the publisher except in the case of brief quotations embodied in critical articles or reviews.

Legal & Disclaimer

The information contained in this book is not designed to replace or take the place of any form of medicine or professional medical advice. The information in this book has been provided for educational and entertainment purposes only.

The information contained in this book has been compiled from sources deemed reliable, and it is accurate to the best of the Author's knowledge; however, the Author cannot guarantee its accuracy and validity and cannot be held liable for any errors or omissions. Changes are periodically made to this book. You must consult your doctor or get professional medical advice before using any of the suggested remedies, techniques, or information in this book.

Table of contents

part 1 1
INTRODUCTION 2
What exactlY is Mediterranean diet? 5
THE ORIGINS OF THE MEDITERRANEAN DIET 8
The Historical Elements of the Mediterranean Diet Scheme 9
The Historical Effects of the Mediterranean Diet Scheme 10
Health benefits of a Mediterranean diet 11
Mediterranean Diet Food PYramid and Food Components ... 12
MYTHS AND FACTS ABOUT THE MEDITERRANEAN DIET 14
Myth 1: It costs a lot to eat this waY. 14
Myth 2: If one glass of wine is good for your heart, then three glasses is three times as healthy 15
Myth 3: Eating large bowls of pasta and bread is the Mediterranean way. 15
Myth 4: The Mediterranean diet is only about the food 16
MEDITERRANEAN DIET FOR DIABETES PREVENTION AND MANAGEMENT 16
MEDITERRANEAN DIET - A HEART HEALTHY DIET 19
Two major benefits are: 20
MEDITERRANEAN DIET FOR WEIGHT LOSS 25
Red meat is eaten in very small amounts in this diet 28
Some more key points to the diet are : 29
Weight Loss Mediterranean Diet Foods 30
MEDITERRANEAN DIET AND DAILY EXERCISE MAINTAIN WEIGHT LOSS 35

MEDITERRANEAN DIET MEAL PLAN AND RECIPES FOR WEIGHT LOSS ... 39

Maple almond granola with coconut ... 40

Spinach and mushroom omelet ... 41

Lebanese hummus ... 42

Lentil soup with olive oil and orange ... 43

Mediterranean baked cod ... 44

Eggplant parmesan with prosciutto ... 45

Hemp and chia seed oatmeal ... 46

Caprese salad skewers ... 47

Easy lemon butter baked fish ... 48

Mediterranean Diet (1 week) Meal Plan for Beginners ... 50

Day 1 ... 50

Breakfast ... 50

Fig & Ricotta Toast ... 50

Lunch ... 51

Green Salad with Pita Bread & Hummus ... 51

Dinner ... 51

Walnut-Rosemary Crusted Salmon ... 52

Day 2 ... 53

Breakfast ... 53

Muesli with Raspberries ... 53

Lunch ... 53

Roasted Veggie & Quinoa Salad ... 53

Dinner ... 54

Tomato & Artichoke Gnocchi ... 54

Day 3 ... 55

Breakfast 55
Creamy Mediterranean Paninis 55
Lunch 56
Tomato & Artichoke Gnocchi 56
Dinner 57
Cod in Tomato Cream Sauce 57
Day 4 58
Breakfast 59
Creamy Blueberry-Pecan Overnight Oats 59
Lunch 59
Roasted Veggie & Hummus Pita Pockets 59
Dinner 60
Chicken & White Bean Soup 60
Day 5 61
Breakfast 61
Muesli with Raspberries 61
Chicken & White Bean Soup 61
Dinner 62
Roasted Root Vegetables with Goat Cheese 62
Vegetables 63
Day 6 64
Breakfast 64
Creamy Blueberry-Pecan Overnight Oats 64
Lunch 64
Chickpea & Veggie Grain Bowl 64
Dinner 65
Mediterranean Chicken & Orzo 65

Day 7 66
Breakfast 66
Rainbow Frittata 66
Lunch 67
Tuna salad 67
Dinner 68
Dijon Salmon with Green Bean Pilaf 68
GREAT MEDITERREAN DIET RECIPES 69
Pasta salad 69
Seafood grill with skordalia 70
Chickpea patties 72
Salmon 73
Shrimp and pasta 74
Portobello mushrooms with mediterranean stuffing 75
Greek-style picnic salad 76
Stuffed tomatoes 78
Breakfast couscous 78
Pizza 79
Grilled vegetable tagine 80
Greek salmon burgers 82
Stuffed roasted red peppers 83
Chicken-garbanzo salad 84
Two-bean greek salad 85
Potato hash with asparagus, chickpeas and poached eggs 87
Israeli pasta salad 89
Cauliflower pizza with greek yogurt pesto & grilled 91
Greek farro salad 93

One pot greek chicken & lemon rice	95
Greek turkey meatball gyro with tzatziki	97
Spinach, feta & artichoke matzo mina	98
Slow cooker mediterranean chicken	101
Greek quesadillas	101
Flatbread pizzas with white bean spinach pesto	103
Chopped salad	104
Toss salad with enough vinaigrette to coat everything. Serve and enjoy	105
Mediterranean nachos	108
Greek super grains salad with homemade pita chips	111
Avgolemono greek lemon chicken soup	112
Salmon souvlaki bowls	113
Smoky vegan moussaka	115
Roasted cabbage steaks with basil pesto & feta	117
Spanish garlic shrimp	118
Quinoa stuffed eggplant with tahini sauce	119
Crock pot chicken thighs with artichokes and sun-dried tomatoes	120
Bowtie pasta with sausage and escarole	122
Spicy greek layered dips	123
Roasted moroccan chicken with spinach salad	124
Whole wheat penne with roasted tomatoes, asparagus, and leeks	125
Farro herb salad with chicken	126
Open-faced chicken bruschetta sandwiches	128
Vegetable lentil soup	129
Spinach feta grilled cheese	130

- Quinoa tabbouleh 132
- Garlic and anchovy roasted lamb chops with a castelvetrano & sage browned butter sauce 133
- Candied grape and cherry tomatoes with baked feta 134
- Walnut-rosemary crusted salmon 135
- Mediterranean Meal Shopping List Ideas 136
- Conclusion 139
- Part 2 143
- INTRODUCTION 144
- CHAPTER ONE 148
- THE LIST OF TRENDING RECIPE 148
- Raitha with cucumber (kheera) 148
- Garlic butter steak bites with zucchini noodles meal prep . 149
- Creamy strawberry-pineapple smoothie 151
- Mango lime smoothie 152
- Coconut oil coffee 153
- CHAPTER tWO 155
- Quick start breakfast drink 155
- Carrot and orange juice 156
- Gingerbread latte syrup 157
- Chocolate- iced mocha 159
- Bowl of oatmeal cookie 160
- Asian noodle salad 161
- Wholewheat spaghetti with sardines and cherry tomatoes 163
- CHAPTER THREE 166
- Salmon pate on wholegrain toast 166
- Flavored latte 167

Okra curry (bhindi or bhinda) 168
Amazing mexican quinoa salad 170
CHAPTER FOUR 174
Warm wild berry buckle from the berry basket 174
Parchment baked salmon 175
Ginger glazed mahi mahi 177
Pesto chicken florentine 178
Black beans and rice 180
CONCLUSION 182

PART 1

INTRODUCTION

In the last few years the Mediterranean region has been the focus of much study; not just for its connections with money and high fashion, but because researchers observed that the region has lesser incidents of heart and chronic diseases. More people there seem to maintain a healthy weight and have a longer lifespan. It's a known fact that obesity is approaching epidemic proportions in the US now, with all its attendant problems and complications.

Perhaps the Mediterranean Diet is what allows people from this region to stay young longer, maintain a healthy weight, a healthy heart and reduce the risk of cancer, hypertension, diabetes, hypercholesterolemia and obesity.

What is the Mediterranean Diet?

It is difficult to come up with an exacting definition of a Mediterranean Diet as the countries in the Mediterranean region consume a diverse set of foods, for example the Spanish consume a healthy amount of fish, olive oil and wine, while the traditional Greek diet consists of 60% fruit and vegetables, 20% meats, 10% carbohydrates and 10% fats.

Characteristically speaking, the Mediterranean diet has high consumption of olive oil. Breads, cereals, fruits and vegetables likewise have a high rate of consumption in the diet. Fish and poultry as well as wine are moderately consumed while eggs and red meat are rated as very low in consumption.

The problem with most diets is that they tend to be extreme. Some diets, like the vegetarian diet, limit a person to just eating fruits, tofu, yogurt and vegetables. Other diets would require high protein intake while severely limiting intake of the other food groups. Like a user friendly computer, the Mediterranean diet does not go to extremes to achieve a desired result. The diet allows for consumption of tasty foods. This allows the dieter to actually enjoy the gastronomic delights normally prohibited by other diets. A solid testament to this fact rests on the presence of wine in the diet.

The most surprising aspect of the Mediterranean diet is that fat is regarded as a healthy dietary component. Keep in mind that it is the fat that gives food most of its flavor. Two substances, omega-3 fatty acids and monounsaturated fats, are considered to be healthy and are not restricted in the diet. Olive oil, canola oil and nuts are good sources of monounsaturated fat while fish, vegetables and nuts contain the healthy omega-3 acids. Saturated fats and trans fat, on the other hand are considered to be unhealthy as they contribute to heart disease. Red meat, butter cheese and milk are sources of saturated fat while processed foods contain hydrogenated oils from which trans fat comes from.

In recent years, a growing number of men and women in different countries around the world have become increasingly concerned about their health. Because of the fact that many people have become more concerned about their overall health, these men and women have paid closer attention to what they eat on a regular basis. In the final analysis, these men and women are making dietary decisions designed to improve their general health and wellbeing.

As people have become more conscious of their health and diet, a considerable number of these same men and women have become interested in the Mediterranean diet regimen. If you are, in fact, a person who appreciates the interrelationship between diet and health, you may have a definite interest in the history of the Mediterranean diet regimen.

Before you can appropriately understand what the Mediterranean diet is all about, you need to appreciate that it is more of a concept than a specific dining routine. In reality, there is no such thing as a Mediterranean diet common to all of the countries in the Mediterranean region of the world. Rather, the "Mediterranean diet" consists of those food items that people who live in the various nations in the region consume in common.

WHAT EXACTLY IS MEDITERRANEAN DIET?

The Mediterranean diet is not a low-fat diet. Fat is actually encouraged, but only healthy varieties such as monounsaturated fat from olive oil and polyunsaturated fat (specifically omega-3 fatty acids) from certain fish and shellfish. Unhealthy fats such as trans fats and saturated fats, which are often found in processed foods and red meat, are discouraged. While the Mediterranean diet is strongly plant-based, it is not exclusively vegetarian. Fish, shellfish, and a little poultry are welcome, but they should never trump whole grains, fruits, vegetables, or legumes in a meal.

Another key component of the Mediterranean diet is lifestyle. Enjoy the social component of eating by sharing meals with family and friends as often as possible, whether on a weeknight or special occasion. Slow down, savor each bite, and don't be afraid to have a glass of wine (or two) in moderation. While wine packs antioxidants, you should also drink plenty of water, as staying properly hydrated keeps your body functioning. The last bit of the equation is making physical activity a part of your daily routine, whether it's biking to work or simply taking a walk during your lunch break to enjoy the fresh air.

In the United States, the Mediterranean diet's popularity continues to rise alongside a growing need for healthier eating patterns and lifestyles. The Centers for Disease Control (CDC) confirms heart disease as the leading cause of death in America for men and women, due to obesity, poor diet, lack of physical activity, diabetes, high levels of bad LDL (low-density lipoprotein) cholesterol, and more. In the 1970s, U.S. physiologist Ancel Keys first linked a Mediterranean-style diet and better cardiovascular health through his "Seven Countries Study," but his theory would not catch on until several decades later. In the 1990s, non-profit Oldways Preservation Trust introduced the Mediterranean Diet pyramid , offering Americans a different approach to healthy eating than the USDA food pyramid provided. Through solid research, increased support from experts, and continued education to the public, the Mediterranean diet is regarded today as a powerful weapon against rising rates of heart disease in the U.S.

The health benefits of the Mediterranean diet are evident from both a medical and holistic perspective. While weight loss is not the primary intent of this diet, it's an inherent effect from eating more plant-based foods while curbing sugar and red meat. Additionally, the high-fiber content of many whole grains, vegetables, fruits, and legumes found in the Mediterranean diet will help you feel fuller for longer, and reduce the chance of overeating. You'll also pick up additional perks such as better digestive health and effective weight management. A Mediterranean diet can also be beneficial to those with type-2 diabetes by helping to lower blood glucose levels while promoting good HDL (high-density lipoprotein) cholesterol. Lastly, studies have also shown a link between the Mediterranean diet and long-term brain health. These health perks, combined with increased exercise and leisure-time, help earn the Mediterranean diet its reputation as a well rounded, logical, and realistic way to live.

The practice of doctors prescribing the Mediterranean diet as a way to reduce the risk of cardiovascular disease is certainly on the rise. We asked top medical experts in the fields of nutrition, epidemiology, and cardiology to share why they advocate a Mediterranean diet:

"The effectiveness of the traditional Mediterranean diet for preventing cardiovascular disease and premature death has been tested by both time and rigorous scientific methods. Health care providers should feel confident recommending this as a way of helping their patients live long and well. ---Walter Willett, MD D.Ph., Professor of Epidemiology and Nutrition at Harvard T.H. Chan School of Public Health

The eating style with the most impressive evidence to support its health benefits is the Mediterranean diet. However, this is not the American version of the Mediterranean diet, which tends to be heavy on pasta, pizza and meat. Instead, it's the traditional peasant Mediterranean diet, whose followers could not afford refined sugar, processed foods, butter and meats. Instead, they grew and ate their own vegetables and berries, and tended orchards of olives, nuts, and fruits. They fished the seas and rivers for their protein, which was rich in omega-3 fats. They consumed modest amounts of fermented dairy such as yogurt and cheese. Many of them during their largest meal of the day would enjoy a glass of red wine from their own vineyards. This diet and lifestyle has been proven in many large studies to be the healthiest eating pattern in the world; and it helps that it is delicious as well as nutritious.

THE ORIGINS OF THE MEDITERRANEAN DIET

The concept of the Mediterranean diet is derived from the eating habits and patterns of the people who populate the countries of Italy, Greece, Spain, France, Tunisia, Lebanon and Morocco. As a result, the Mediterranean diet actually includes a tremendous array of delectable food. In point of fact, if a person elects to adopt the concept of the Mediterranean dining scheme, or if a person elects to follow a Mediterranean diet regimen, he or she will have the ability to enjoy a remarkable assortment of scrumptious fare.

The diet of the peoples that have populated the regions around the Mediterranean Sea actually have remained nearly completely unchanged for well over one thousand years. The history of the region is replete with examples of men and women living longer than similarly situated people who consumed alternate diets. Through the centuries, the people of the Mediterranean Sea region have enjoyed longer lives that people in other parts of the world at the same historical epoch.

At the heart of the Mediterranean diet are foods and beverages that are indigenous to the geographic landmass surrounding the Mediterranean Sea. In short, the development of the Mediterranean dieting and dining pattern initially developed by providence. The people of the region naturally and understandably ate those foods and drank those beverages that readily were available in and around their homes.

The Historical Elements of the Mediterranean Diet Scheme

As mentioned previously, over the centuries, the diet of the peoples of the Mediterranean Sea region has remained essentially unchanged. The Mediterranean diet consists of the bountiful consumption of a number of healthy food items including:

- Fresh fruit
- Fresh vegetables
- Low fat nuts
- Whole grains
- Monounsaturated fat

In a similar vein, the Mediterranean diet utilized by people for generation after generation excludes or limits certain food items that have been deemed harmful in recent scientific studies. These less than desirable food items include:

- Saturated fats
- Red and fatty meat
- Rich dairy products
- Fatty fish

THE HISTORICAL EFFECTS OF THE MEDITERRANEAN DIET SCHEME

As has been alluded to earlier in this book on the history of the Mediterranean diet regimen, the people who inhabit the region have a demonstrably lower rate of heart disease and related ailments that oftentimes have a direct dietary connection. With the advent of scientific studies that have correlated the incidence of health problems with a poor diet, the positive effects of the Mediterranean diet have become self evident.

Research over the course of the past two decades has conclusively demonstrated that the men and women who populate the Mediterranean region are afflicted with heart disease and similar ailments far less often than people in other regions of the world. The experts who have conducted these studies have concluded that there is a strong likelihood that the diet scheme that is common in the Mediterranean region is responsible for maintaining the good health of the people who live in that corner of the globe throughout the past one thousand years.

Health benefits of a Mediterranean diet

A traditional Mediterranean diet consisting of large quantities of fresh fruits and vegetables, nuts, fish and olive oil, coupled with physical activity can reduce your risk of serious mental and physical health problems by:

Preventing heart disease and strokes. Following a Mediterranean diet limits your intake of refined breads, processed foods, and red meat, and encourages drinking red wine instead of hard liquor all factors that can help prevent heart disease and stroke.

Keeping you agile. If you're an older adult, the nutrients gained with a Mediterranean diet may reduce your risk of developing muscle weakness and other signs of frailty by about 70 percent.

Reducing the risk of Alzheimer's. Research suggests that the Mediterranean diet may improve cholesterol, blood sugar levels, and overall blood vessel health, which in turn may reduce your risk of Alzheimer's disease or dementia.

Halving the risk of Parkinson's disease. The high levels of antioxidants in the Mediterranean diet can prevent cells from undergoing a damaging process called oxidative stress, thereby cutting the risk of Parkinson's disease in half.

Increasing longevity. By reducing your risk of developing heart disease or cancer with the Mediterranean diet, you're reducing your risk of death at any age by 20%.

Protecting against type 2 diabetes. A Mediterranean diet is rich in fiber which digests slowly, prevents huge swings in blood sugar, and can help you maintain a healthy weight.

MEDITERRANEAN DIET FOOD PYRAMID AND FOOD COMPONENTS

Plant-based foods such as whole grains, vegetables, fruits, legumes, nuts, and seeds, and healthy fats such as olive oil should be worked into every meal when possible. Below, we break down six essential components of the Mediterranean diet.

1. **Healthy Grains:** Whether enjoyed for breakfast, lunch, or dinner, whole, healthy grains are full of fiber, antioxidants, and anti-inflammatory properties. A 2015 study in JAMA Internal Medicine linked whole grains and lower mortality, especially from chronic diseases such as cardiovascular disease and type-2 diabetes. Common whole grains include brown rice and oats, while ancient grains such as quinoa, amaranth, farro, buckwheat, and bulgur pack the added perk of being gluten-free.

2. **Vegetables:** These plant-based foods are colorful, nutritious, and extremely versatile. Whether raw, grilled, steamed, sautéed, roasted, or pickled, vegetables should be on your plate during every meal. They're easy to spread over pizza, mix into scrambled eggs, or toss into salads.

3. **Proteins:** Good proteins to eat include fish and shellfish, especially varieties packing omega-3 fatty acids. Some of the healthiest seafood you can eat are salmon, arctic char, mackerel, anchovies, and oysters. Don't forget about plant proteins such as beans, legumes, nuts, and seeds—these foods contain unsaturated fats, fiber, and can add instant texture and flavor to salads or stand alone as satisfying snacks.

4. **Fruits:** Healthy fruits in the Mediterranean diet include olives, avocados, grapes, and figs, all of which pack fiber and antioxidants. Consume as many types of fruit as possible from seasonal to locally grown. In

terms of when to eat fruit, focus on when you would normally crave a sugar fix such as in the afternoon or after dinner.

5. **Healthy Fats**: Olive oil is the primary healthy fat of the Mediterranean diet and is used for cooking, baking, sauces, vinaigrettes, and more. In addition to olive oil, the American Heart Association recommends healthy cooking oils such as canola, peanut, and safflower.

6. **Red Wine:** The health benefits of red wine are particular noteworthy. A 2015 study published in the Annals of Internal Medicine linked one serving of red wine daily (150ml. or 5 oz.) to an increase of good cholesterol in the body. Sipping a glass of wine can help you de-stress while also enhancing the flavor of your food.

MYTHS AND FACTS ABOUT THE MEDITERRANEAN DIET

Following a Mediterranean diet has many benefits, but there are still a lot of misconceptions on exactly how to take advantage of the lifestyle to lead a healthier, longer life. The following are some myths and facts about the Mediterranean diet.

MYTH 1: IT COSTS A LOT TO EAT THIS WAY.

Fact: If you're creating meals out of beans or lentils as your main source of protein, and sticking with mostly plants and whole grains, then the Mediterranean diet is less expensive than serving dishes of packaged or processed foods.

MYTH 2: IF ONE GLASS OF WINE IS GOOD FOR YOUR HEART, THEN THREE GLASSES IS THREE TIMES AS HEALTHY.

Fact: Moderate amounts of red wine (one drink a day for women; two for men) certainly has unique health benefits for your heart, but drinking too much has the opposite effect. Anything more than two glasses of wine can actually be bad for your heart.

MYTH 3: EATING LARGE BOWLS OF PASTA AND BREAD IS THE MEDITERRANEAN WAY.

Fact: Typically, Mediterraneans don't eat a huge plate of pasta the way Americans do. Instead, pasta is usually a side dish with about a 12-cup to 1-cup serving size. The rest of their plate consists of salads, vegetables, fish or a small portion of organic, grass-fed meat, and perhaps one slice of bread.

MYTH 4: THE MEDITERRANEAN DIET IS ONLY ABOUT THE FOOD.

Fact: The food is a huge part of the diet, yes, but don't overlook the other ways the Mediterraneans live their lives. When they sit down for a meal, they don't sit in front of a television or eat in a rush; they sit down for a relaxed, leisurely meal with others, which may be just as important for your health as what's on your plate. Mediterraneans also enjoy plenty of physical activity.

MEDITERRANEAN DIET FOR DIABETES PREVENTION AND MANAGEMENT

You may think of heart health when you think of a Mediterranean diet, but this eating pattern can help with blood sugar, too. People who follow a Mediterranean diet are less likely to develop type 2 diabetes. People with diabetes who follow this diet pattern can have lower blood sugar and glycated hemoglobin, and reduced insulin resistance. The diet is even linked to fewer diabetes complications.

The heart-healthy benefits of a Mediterranean diet can be even more important in diabetes because having diabetes puts you at risk for high blood pressure and cardiovascular disease. Not surprisingly, the diet pattern lowers cardiovascular risk in patients with diabetes. People with diabetes who follow a Mediterranean diet pattern may have a lower risk for peripheral arterial disease and other cardiovascular conditions, as well as lower blood pressure and lower mortality rates. It can have anti-inflammatory effects, which means it can lower risk of other chronic conditions.

When it comes to living with diabetes, a low carb, Mediterranean style diet has been shown to be more effective than the typical calorie restricted, low-fat eating plan according to a just-released study appearing in the September 1st issue of the Annals of Internal Medicine looking at the recommended diet for diabetes sufferers.

Until now both of these eating plans had been recommended for weight loss in overweight (or obese) patients diagnosed with type 2 diabetes, but there have been few direct comparisons of the eating plans.

Seeing this and wanting to asses the effectiveness, durability and safety of the two diets, Dr. Dario Giugliano of the Second University of Naples in Italy and his team randomly assigned 215 subjects with newly diagnosed type 2 diabetes who had never treated with medication to either a low carb Mediterranean style diet or a low-fat diet.

This was a lifestyle, not a fat diet tried on for a few weeks. Both groups received monthly counseling sessions from nutritionists and dietitians for the first year, every other month for the remaining three years.

At the end of the four year study, one of the longest running of its kind, 44% of those on the Mediterranean style diet needed medication to lower their blood sugar, compared to 70% needing medication from the low-fat diet group.

At the one-year mark, subjects following the Mediterranean diet lost more weight - a difference of 4.4 pounds. These dieters also had slimmer waistlines. This group even saw greater increases in HDL (good) cholesterol and bigger decreases in harmful triglycerides. The heart healthy benefits remained for the duration of the study.

Understand there's no one "Mediterranean" diet, at least 16 countries all with their own tastes combine to create the eating plan that's taken on the name. It's best to think of the Mediterranean diet as a way of living and eating that all about plenty of fruits, vegetables, fish and whole grains, with limits on red meat and processed foods.

Fat come from olive and canola oils as well as small portions of nuts such as walnuts, pecans, almonds and hazelnuts. Herbs and spices (not salt) are used to flavor foods. Carbs are few. Red wine, in moderation (5 ounces daily for women or men over age 65, no more than 10 ounces daily for men under age 65) is in there too.

But it's not all about food; the Mediterranean diet is also about eating meals with family and friends. The chance to socialize and enjoy companionship as well as food.

The low fat diet used in the research was based on the American Heart Association guidelines. It had lots of whole grains, limited sweets and allowed no more than 30% of calories to come from fat, keeping to 10% from saturated (animal) fats.

If this type of eating plan is working for you, this latest study isn't any reason to change your eating plan, but you can be aware, so you're making an informed decision about your diet plan.

What's worrisome for the medical community is that the numbers with type 2 diabetes is growing quickly, with an estimated 380 million cases by 2025

Today diabetes affects over 20 million Americans and brings symptoms like blurred vision, fatigue, increased appetite, thirst and need to urinate. Since type 2 diabetes develops slowly, some people don't experience many symptoms.

MEDITERRANEAN DIET - A HEART HEALTHY DIET

Cretans from the Greek island of Crete and other Greeks live longer than many other populations in the world. They are 20% less likely to die of coronary artery heart disease than the people living in North America. Along with populations of southern Italy, they also enjoy a significant decrease in the incidence of chronic diseases. This health bonanza has been attributed primarily to their diet. In 2002, Curtis and O'Keefe in the Postgraduate Journal, suggested that the Mediterranean Diet could be the new 'Gold Standard' for heart disease prevention. (Curtis B, O'Keefe J. Understanding the Mediterranean Diet: Could This Be the New "Gold Standard" for Heart Disease Prevention? Postgraduate Medicine. 2002; 112(2):35-8.). These populations have an unique dietary tradition - they regularly use liberal amounts of olive oil, nuts, grains, beans, fruits and vegetables in their food. They also eat fish regularly and indulge in moderate amount of wine drinking. Their diet is limited in red meat, refined grains, sugars and processed food items. The effects include an improvement in lipid profile, reduction in blood pressure, decrease in insulin resistance and induces favorable changes in the markers of inflammation - leading to decreased heart disease.

As mentioned above, adherence to the Mediterranean diet also protects against several chronic diseases. (Gjonça A, Bobak M. Albanian Paradox.)

TWO MAJOR BENEFITS ARE:

Decrease in the risk of developing diabetes mellitus: M Á Martínez-González and associates followed 13 380 Spanish university graduates without diabetes at baseline followed them for a median of 4.4 years. They found that those who adhered to the Mediterranean diet had a lower risk of developing diabetes. (M Á Martínez-González, C de la Fuente-Arrillaga, J M Nunez-Cordoba et al. Adherence to Mediterranean diet and risk of developing diabetes: prospective cohort study. BMJ 2008;336:1348-1351). The benefits accrued from decreases in insulin resistance and increases in insulin sensitivity. Mediterranean diet is also inversely associated with the metabolic syndrome - a key risk factor associated with the development of diabetes.

Decrease in cancer: In 2004 Trichopoulou noted that one reason for the increase in longevity in people following the Mediterranean diet was a reduction in the incidence of cancer. (Trichopoulou A, Critselis E. Mediterranean diet and longevity. European Journal of Cancer Prevention. 2004;13(5):453-6.). A recent report has again verified these findings (Benetou V, Trichopoulou A, Orfanos P. Conformity to traditional Mediterranean diet and cancer incidence: the Greek EPIC cohort. British Journal of Cancer. 2008;99:191-5.). The cancer risk can be cut by almost 12% by just adding a few elements of the Mediterranean diet to the western diet - reducing red meat intake and increasing the intake of peas, beans, lentils and olive oil. Scientists reached this conclusion after monitoring the detailed dietary records of over 26,000 Greek men and women, over a period of eight years.

Other benefits noted and well documented in clinical studies include improvement in Alzhiemer's disease, Parkinsons disease, rheumatoid arthritis, depression and body weight. This was recently confirmed again in a study by Sofi and associates and published in the British Medical Journal of 12 September, 2008.

It stands to logic that the reduction in chronic diseases, especially heart ailments, diabetes and cancer should lead to an increased longevity. And the data has supported this:

The people of the Mediterranean region enjoy a flavorful and healthy diet. Traditional foods from countries like Algeria, Cyprus, Egypt, France, Greece, Italy, Libya, Malta, Morocco, Portugal and Spain are low in saturated fat and high in fiber. Various reports have suggested that heart disease rates and deaths from heart attacks are lower in Mediterranean countries than in the United States. The heart health of the Mediterranean people may be due in part to diet and in part to more physical exercise. Adopting a Mediterranean diet and getting more exercise may help reduce your risk of developing heart disease.

The Mediterranean diet consists of fruits, vegetables, potatoes, beans, nuts, seeds and grains like bread. Olive oil is used to prepare these foods. Wine is served with most meals, and red meats and eggs are rare in the Mediterranean diet. Dairy, chicken and fish are eaten occasionally. Begin to transform your diet to be more Mediterranean in makeup and flavor by replacing vegetable, corn and canola oils with olive oil. Don't use butter or margarine either, instead dip flavorful breads in warm olive oil. Vegetables are low in calories, high in fiber and loaded with beneficial antioxidants. Try some Greek vegetarian dishes a few times each week. Greek food is flavorful and healthy.

Cut red meat out of your diet, or consume red meat no more than once each month. Vegetables are the staple foods in a Mediterranean diet. It may be difficult to break old eating habits, but numerous studies indicate that eating a Mediterranean diet can reduce the overall risk of death from heart attack. Red meat is bad for your heart, because it is filled with saturated fat. The Mediterranean diet does not include steaks and ground beef. Beef is eaten rarely and should be as lean as possible. You can replace ground beef with ground turkey burgers on whole wheat buns to help wean you off the red meat. Instead of mayonnaise, pickles, mustard and ketchup, add a slice of tomato, avocado and lettuce to a turkey burger. Changing your diet may contribute to a longer, healthier life.

Replace the white bread in your breadbox with whole grain bread. Refined wheat products, such as white bread and pasta, are high in fat and low in fiber content. Whole grain foods like cereals are rich in vitamins and minerals not found in unfortified refined wheat products. Fish and chicken contain healthy omega-3 fatty acids, which are good for heart health. They are also an ideal source of low-fat protein. Fish and chicken in the Mediterranean diet is usually broiled or baked, but never fried. There are no fried foods in the Mediterranean diet.

Increase in life span: Knoops and associates studied 1,507 healthy men and 832 healthy women aged 70-90 years in 11 European countries (including Italy, Finland, and the Netherlands) between 1988 and 2000. They found that maintaining a Mediterranean diet and a healthy lifestyle resulted in a more than 50% lower risk of death for people 70-90 years old. (Knoops K, de Groot L, Kromhout D, et al: Mediterranean Diet, Lifestyle Factors, and 10-year Mortality in Elderly European Men and Women. The HALE Project. JAMA 292:1433-1439, 2004.) Recent data from a study from Northern Europe shows that this diet also reduces mortality in younger people. (Lagiou P, Trichopoulos D, Sandin S, et al. Mediterranean dietary pattern and mortality among young women: a cohort study in Sweden. British Journal of Nutrition. 2006;96(2):384-92.) The reduction appears to be due to several factors, including reductions in cancer and cardiovascular deaths.

To summarize, healthy 'Mediterranean' food advice is:

- Eat less red meat.
- Consume less milk and dairy products like cream and cheese.
- Eat more fish, especially cold water fish.

- Switch to olive oil.
- Eat more grains, seed and nuts.
- Avoid refined grains and processed foods.
- Eat more fruits and vegetables and legumes.
- And drink alcohol moderately, especially red wine with meals.

MEDITERRANEAN DIET FOR WEIGHT LOSS

Would you be surprised to learn that eating the Mediterranean diet way is not only a healthy way to eat but is an effective and natural way to combat heart disease and some cancers, while losing weight in the process?

For many women, dieting for weight loss can be a daunting and somewhat restricting undertaking and especially so, if you're a vegetarian. Most weight loss diets will nearly always involve giving up or limiting your intake of some of the foods you particularly enjoy. Whether it is a low carb diet such as the atkins diet or any of the many fad diets. Either way you'll most certainly have to deprive yourself in some way. Any diet that involves deprivation in any way shape or form, will lessen your chances of achieving your weight loss diet goals. You're also more likely to regain any lost weight once you've finished your diet and resume normal eating. This is where the Mediterranian diet approach is a god-send.

The Mediterranean diet and lifestyle is being touted as the best two- pronged approach to achieving healthy eating and weight maintenance, without the need to resort to starvation diets or, extra gruelling physical exercise.

This diet consist of mainly fruits, vegetables, beans, potatoes and nuts. The twist to this diet is that meat is not consumed that often as compared to the American diet which is usually very high in saturated fats. This is the main reason for our obesity problem.

Making the switch from your routine diet to a healthier one is a lot easier than you think. You can learn more about how to plan meals in the Mediterranean diet.

Keep in mind that it is by no means a strict meal plan. It will always be to your advantage to follow a meal plan that works for you so be certain to explore your option and design a personal meal plan you will stick to.

It is very much possible to lose weight under the Mediterranean diet. For better results though, you want to consult your dietitian for the best meal plan for this purpose. Remember that this diet calls for increased physical activity as well. You will need time to lie down, rest and relax too.

You will notice that beverages such as alcohol or coffee are not included in this meal plan. These exclusions are based on the Mediterranean meal plan and are considered optional at best. What you drink during meals in entirely up to you. Be sure to base this decision on your current overall health though.

As a healthier alternative, consider making Green Tea part of your diet. This drink has plenty of health benefits for you. Caffeine and alcoholic drinks should be taken in moderation. This is especially true if you are trying to lose weight.

Recipes for the dishes included in this meal plan can be found in the next chapter. When making a meal plan, keep these guidelines in mind:

o Enjoy your food.- Remember that relishing every flavor of your food is part of the Mediterranean way of life. Beyond good nutrition, eating is a feast for the senses you must enjoy. It is not considered an inconvenient chore but an important part of life.

o Watch the servings.- In any diet, it is important for your calorie intake and activity level to break even. For weight loss, you want to consume fewer calories and move around more. Of course this is easier said than done in today's lifestyle. Again, it is important to ask for advice from a dietitian or other nutrition expert. In this meal plan, it is up to you to adjust serving sizes to meet your needs.

o Drink plenty of water.- As much as possible, try to drink at least six to eight glasses of water a day.

o Exercise, rest and relax- Apart from the diet itself, what you do in between meals is an important part of the Mediterranean diet. You should spend less time sitting down and more time moving and getting around. Go outdoors and find something to do to cover your exercise. Be sure to get enough rest and relaxation as well.

RED MEAT IS EATEN IN VERY SMALL AMOUNTS IN THIS DIET

Maybe this iswhy people from this region have much lower cases of heart disease and weight problems. It's the kind of diet that is worth taking a look at. One of the main problems here in America is that we just consume way too much meat and highly saturated fatty foods that do nothing but clog your arteries and cause massive heart attacks.

You may be asking, how do you add flavor to the Mediterranean diet? The main ingredient that they use to add flavor to the food is olive oil, which is healthy and it adds a good light flavor to the food. Their has been a study put together that prove that people that ate the diet will actually cut their risk of heart disease by a whopping 25 percent!

If you have never tried the Mediterranean food, you will be in for a treat. The great thing that I like about this kind of food is that it's very light. You have the feeling of being full, but not the heavy bloated feeling that no one really likes. If you are a big eater you can modify the diet to fit your taste and still benefit from it.

The diet has a distinctive taste that I think you will love.

SOME MORE KEY POINTS TO THE DIET ARE :

- Eggs are consumed no more than 3 times per week
- Wine is consumed because of its antioxidant properties
- Most people go on the Mediterranean diet to lose weight

Do you think the diet is something that is worth giving a shot? This is one of the rare natural diets that will help you lose weight. Give it a try! You will be pleasantly surprised by the taste.

It is as the name suggests, a diet typical for people living in the Mediterranean would eat. This means a diet high in fruits and vegetables as well as beans, lentils and legumes. It also incorporates healthy fats and avoids saturated fats from fatty meats and unhealthy dairy products that contribute to bad cholesterol.

WEIGHT LOSS MEDITERRANEAN DIET FOODS

High Amounts of Healthy Carbohydrates - Wholegrain breads, pasta, Brown Rice, couscous, Polenta and Sweet Potato (regular potato's are OK but contain little nutrients and have quite a large impact on blood sugar)

High Amounts of Fruits - 3-5 pieces of fruit and vegetables a day. Try and choose a variety of fruits and vegetables and not always eat the same kinds.

Moderate Amounts of Steamed and grilled fish

Moderate amounts of olive oil- the Mediterranean diet foods include extra virgin olive oil and it's recommended that you pour the olive oil onto your foods raw and avoid cooking as it cooking the oil makes breaks it down into a less healthier form.

Small Amounts of lean red meat- when eating meat choose lean cuts of meat with very little visible fat.

Small amounts of alcohol are allowed- Small amounts of wine are popular on the the diet

High Amount of Anti-oxidants- The diet incorporates a large amount of anti-oxidants which you will absorb through the fresh fruit and vegetables you consume.

The Mediterranean diet is the name that has been given to a particular dietary regimen that was originally used by people in poorer regions of Italy and Greece for many centuries. This diet was not originally thought to be particularly healthy in these regions, as the people ate these foods because of necessity, rather than because of the Mediterranean diet weight loss and excellent nutrition benefits they experienced. This type of cuisine is far different from what you might expect from this region, but it is overall much healthier because things like lard and butter are rarely used.

Basically, a Mediterranean diet calls for people to eat a great deal of fresh fruit, plant foods, fish, poultry, some dairy products, while using extra virgin olive oil as the primary source of fat. Also, a moderate amount of eggs can be eaten each month, while red meat is to be avoided as much as possible. Red meat can be eaten in low amounts, but meals should not be centered around it because of how it affects the heart. The Mediterranean diet is meant to lower the risk of heart disease, since olive oil is high in monounsaturated fats, which have been known to reduce this risk substantially. This also reduces the body's cholesterol levels, which is also a positive thing for the body.

Even though this diet was first brought to light in 1945, it did not really hit mainstream levels until the 1990s, when people began to develop a newfound awareness of what they were eating. This is around the time that exercise shows began appearing on television and healthy eating began to become popular again. The

Mediterranean diet is based on the idea that people in these regions have a much lower rate of heart disease than people with similar fat intake in other areas of the world. For example, a person living in the United States and a person living in Greece could consume the exact same amount of fat year after year, but the American would have a higher chance of suffering from heart disease because he or she is missing certain elements from his or her diet.

The main ingredient in a Mediterranean diet that is believed to have the most influence on a person's health is extra virgin olive oil. This is because the diet is inherently low in saturated fat, but the olive oil makes it high in monounsaturated fat, which (as previously mentioned) is good for your heart. The Mediterranean diet is also very high in dietary fiber, which promotes regularity of the digestive system. The diet can sometimes be high in salt, when is contains:

Olives

Capers

Salad dressing

Fish roe

This salt content is not necessarily a negative thing however, because those items contain natural salts the body can use and absorb more comfortably.

One thing that many people might not realize about Mediterranean diet weight loss is that the people who originated the diet generally worked outdoors and reaonably hard. This means they were getting plenty of exercise each and every day, in addition to fresh air. This, in combination with the small portions these individuals would eat, led to very lean and muscular bodies. This assisted heart health of course, which is another reason why they suffered far fewer deaths from cardiovascular problems.

A number of medical studies have been conducted on the Mediterranean diet and they have found that men who lived in Crete, which is one of the regions where this diet was originally used, had a low incidence of heart disease. This occurred despite the fact they actually consumed high amounts of fats in many cases. One of the main reasons for this finding is that many of these men switched from butter to extra virgin olive oil because it was less expensive. They also had a high vitamin C intake and reduced the amount of red meat compared to other parts of the globe. It should be noted that the findings of this study were so dramatic that the results were published before the study had been completed. This was because the people who were conducting the study did not believe they could keep the information to themselves any longer. Other diseases and illnesses which have been positively affected from this diet include osteoporosis, minimising the risk of some forms of cancer, allergies, alzheimers disease and there are more studies being undertaken.

Further studies have shown instances of Mediterranean diet weight loss, as 322 people participated in an experiment where some people were subject to a low-carb diet, others undertook a low-fat diet, and some ate only a Mediterranean diet. The results showed that those who were on the Mediterranean diet had the greatest weight loss of all, with the top two participants losing 12 and 10 pounds respectively. The study highlighted that Mediterranean diet weight loss is effective and should be considered by anyone who is having trouble losing weight.

The Mediterranean diet is not just a way to lose weight, but is a way to entirely change your life, and in doing so, helping to prolong it. The health benefits are endless, especially when they are combined with exercise, making this nutrition adventure something definitely worth looking into. The bottom line is - those who are on this diet have lower mortality rates than those who are not, which is reason enough to give it a try. If you have a history of heart disease in your family, you really cannot afford to continue the same path and now you have an alternative.

MEDITERRANEAN DIET AND DAILY EXERCISE MAINTAIN WEIGHT LOSS

Healthy living is a treasured wealth that does not come on its own. It has to be planned. Food plays a vital role in providing essential nutrients for growth and development of the body. While some foods are considered healthy and are required in large quantities, others may be exempt from a daily diet. This is how a Mediterranean diet plan works.

The Mediterranean diet is considered to be the most suitable form of healthy diet. Researchers have proved that the secret of healthy living of people in the Mediterranean region can be attributed to their balanced diet and active life style. Studies have also shown that this diet not only lowers chronic heart diseases but also improves life expectancy.

The Mediterranean diet is considered to be the most suitable form of healthy dieting. Researchers have proved that the secret of healthy living of people in the Mediterranean region can be attributed to their balanced diet and active life style. Studies have also shown that this diet not only lowers chronic heart diseases but also improves life expectancy

Doctors frequently advise obese patients, particularly those with metabolic syndrome, to lose weight by adopting a healthy lifestyle. While low-fat and low-carb diets help in the short-term, research doesn't support their long-term benefits. A new study found the combination of the Mediterranean diet and exercise promoted weight loss and reduced cardiovascular risk, benefits that were maintained after one year.

In the research published in the journal Diabetes Care, scientists studied 626 overweight patients between the ages of 55 and 75. The participants had at least three of the following cardiovascular risk factors: high blood pressure, abdominal obesity, high blood sugar levels, low HDL cholesterol and high triglycerides. Researchers monitored changes in fat accumulation, body weight and an array of cardiovascular risk indicators throughout 12 months.

The results showed that consumption of the Mediterranean diet, which is naturally low in calories, led to at least a five-percent weight reduction. In addition, the participants experienced improvements in inflammatory markers and glucose metabolism compared to those who didn't follow the diet. Moreover, patients who had diabetics or a risk of diabetes enjoyed especially high glucose control benefits.

According to the research team, the most weight loss was noted after 12 months, a finding that shows the weight reduction was maintained over time. They concluded that the Mediterranean diet and a regular exercise program may produce long-term advantages for cardiovascular disease, which would translate into fewer deaths from heart attacks and strokes.

Nowadays, overweight or obese patients, particularly those with metabolic syndrome, are recommended to lose weight by changing their lifestyle. The aim of these recommendations is to reduce their cardiovascular risk; however, there is no scientific evidence that this beneficial effect can be maintained in the long-term. Although low fat and low carbohydrate diets have proven effective in losing weight and improving cardiovascular risk, the benefits tend to diminish after a year.

With this investigation, the researchers from the Human Nutrition Unit at the Universitat Rovira i Virgili, in collaboration with 23 other research groups in the PREDIMED-Plus study, have evaluated the changes in body weight, fat accumulation and different cardiovascular risk factors after one year in 626 patients. The results have shown that the lifestyle changes included in the study are effective in maintain clinically significant weight loss. Indeed, after 12 months of intervention, 33.7% of the patients following the hypocaloric Mediterranean diet and daily exercise showed a minimum of 5% weight loss. These patients also showed improvements in those parameters related with glucose metabolism and certain inflammatory markers, in contrast with those patients who did not follow the diet. Furthermore, for those patients with diabetes or at risk of diabetes, the benefits from these lifestyle changes were particularly high in terms of glucose control.

The researchers highlight that, in this study, the greatest weight loss has been found after 12 months, which illustrates that weight loss was maintained over time.

"Fad diets like low-carb diets allow people to lose weight quickly, but we need to look at their sustainability and their impact on long-term health. Such diets are hard to follow over a long period, and they carry cardiovascular risks. This is why, as a cardiologist, I prefer the Mediterranean diet, which can be used from the very young to the very old. It's the ideal eating pattern because it promotes weight management, along with multiple other wellness benefits.

"The Mediterranean diet has been researched extensively. Studies show it reduces the likelihood of cardiovascular disease, Alzheimer's disease, blood clots and metabolic syndrome. The evidence also indicates the diet improves insulin sensitivity, lowers oxidative stress, decreases inflammation and enhances endothelial cell function.

"Consumption of the toxic American diet, which is calorie-dense, nutrient-depleted and highly processed, leads to many medical problems. Conversely, the unprocessed foods that comprise the Mediterranean diet provide the body with nutrients it needs to maximize health. It's rich in fruits, vegetables, legumes, fatty fish, nuts, seeds and extra virgin olive oil. The eating plan is also low in red meat and sugary beverages.

"Combining the Mediterranean diet with exercise can do much to prevent disease. By Michael Ozner, a board-certified cardiologist, specializing in heart disease prevention, and author of The Complete Mediterranean Diet.

MEDITERRANEAN DIET MEAL PLAN AND RECIPES FOR WEIGHT LOSS

A modified Mediterranean Diet meal plan has been shown to help people lose weight and most importantly, to keep the weight off. I personally have lost 40 pounds eating the Mediterranean Diet and have been able to keep the weight off for 2 years. The trick, for me, has been losing the weight slowly and only having to modify my diet slightly. When I want to lose weight, I eat a modified Mediterranean diet, which for me, means eating gluten and sugar free. This, along with exercising, eating only fruit after dinner and watching my portion sizes will do the trick. The best part is that I know this is only temporary while I lose the weight. I can easily maintain my weight and eat gluten and some sugar. During weight loss I still eat everything else Mediterranean including lots of olive oil, fruits and vegetables, beans, nuts, seeds, some meat and non-glutenous whole grains such as rice, quinoa, corn, millet and oats. The food is delicious and losing weight is less of a struggle and more of a culinary journey.

Below is a collection of Mediterranean Diet recipes that are helpful for weight loss. If you eat a true Mediterranean diet you can still lose weight even if many of your calories are coming from extra virgin olive oil. Olive oil will help fill you up so you are less likely to crave processed foods and sugars.

What you will find with these easy recipes, is that Mediterranean food is so delicious and filling, you won't feel like you're on a diet.

MAPLE ALMOND GRANOLA WITH COCONUT

Ingredients

- 3 cups old fashioned oats (gluten free)

- 1 cup sliced almonds
- ¾ cup shredded coconut
- ¼ cup brown sugar
- ¼ cup of olive oil
- ¼ cup maple syrup
- ¾ teaspoon salt

Direction

Preheat oven to 250 degrees Fahrenheit.

In a large mixing bowl, mix together oats, almonds, coconut, and brown sugar.

In a small mixing bowl, mix together olive oil, maple syrup, and salt.

Add liquid to dry ingredients. Stir until everything is incorporated well.

Spread granola evenly over two cookie sheets. Bake for 1 hour and 15 minutes, stirring every 15 minutes until granola is golden brown and crispy.

SPINACH AND MUSHROOM OMELET

Ingredients

- 2 tsps extra virgin olive oil
- 2 cups mushrooms, sliced
- 1 onion, chopped

- 4 cups spinach, stems removed if needed
- 4 eggs, whisked
- salt and pepper, to taste
- 1 tsp dried oregano

Direction

In a non-stick pan, heat 1 tsp of olive oil on medium heat. Add mushroom and onions.

Saute mushrooms and onions for 3 minutes then add spinach.

Season with salt, pepper, and oregano.

Once cooked to desired tenderness, remove the vegetables from the pan.

Keep pan on medium heat. Add tsp of remaining olive oil and pour in whipped eggs. Sprinkle with a little more oregano, salt, and pepper.

Top one side of omelet with cooked veggies. Fold omelet over with a spatula. Cook until eggs are done.

LEBANESE HUMMUS

Ingredients

- 2 -15 oz cans chickpeas, drained and rinsed
- 2 garlic cloves, crushed
- 14 cup tahini paste

- 13 cup freshly squeezed lemon juice
- 14 cup extra virgin olive oil
- 14 tsp paprika
- 12 tsp salt
- 3 tbsp cold water
- pine nuts for garnish (optional)

Direction

Begin by chopping the garlic in the food processor.

Add the rest of the ingredients and blend in the food processor until desired consistency.

Blend with cold water for a smoother consistency.

LENTIL SOUP WITH OLIVE OIL AND ORANGE

Ingredients

- 1 pound lentils, washed well, stones removed
- 6 cups water
- 1 cup extra virgin olive oil
- 2 cloves garlic, minced
- 2 tablespoons tomato paste
- 1 onion, grated
- 3 carrots, grated
- 2 orange slices, peel and flesh
- 1 bay leaf
- Salt and pepper, to taste

Direction

In a deep pot, add lentils and 6 cups water. Bring to a boil and continue boiling for 15 minutes.

Add remaining ingredients and continue cooking on a low boil for 30 minutes or until lentils are soft. Add more water if needed.

MEDITERRANEAN BAKED COD

Ingredients

- 4 cod filets (1 12 lbs total)
- 12 tsp salt
- 12 cup lemon juice
- 1 Tbsp Dijon mustard
- 2 onions, sliced thin
- 2 fresh tomatoes, diced
- 2 cloves garlic, minced
- 14 cup capers, drained
- 12 tsp pepper
- 2 Tbsp rosemary, dried or fresh
- 14 cup extra virgin olive oil

Direction

Preheat oven to 350 degrees F. Sprinkle salt on cod filets.

Whisk together lemon juice and mustard in a small bowl.

Prepare 4 pieces of parchment paper as done in video.

Put a small handful of onions near the middle of the parchment paper, next to the fold. Place a cod filet on top. Repeat for each filet.

Layer chopped tomatoes, onion, minced garlic, capers, pepper, and rosemary on top of each cod filet.

Spoon on 14 of the lemonmustard mixture and a Tablespoon of olive oil on each filet.

Close packet by folding edges and overlapping

Bake at 350 F for 15 minutes for perfectly flaky fish.

Eggplant Parmesan with Prosciutto

Ingredients
- 1 Cup tomato sauce
- 2 medium sized eggplants
- 6 ounces of thinly sliced, raw Parma Ham (Prosciutto)
- Olive oil
- Butter
- Salt and pepper to taste
- 1 Cup grated Parmesan cheese

Direction

Gently simmer the tomato sauce.

Trim the eggplant and cut into rounds; Sprinkle the eggplant with salt and place in a colander for 20 minutes; Rinse slices and pat dry.

Heat a generous layer of olive oil in a frying pan and fry the eggplant slices on both slides until they are golden, then dry on paper towels.

Place a layer of the eggplant slices at the bottom of a well-buttered baking dish, cover with slices of ham, a few tablespoons of tomato sauce, pepper, and generously sprinkle with Parmesan cheese. Repeat the layers until the ingredients are all used.

Dot the surface with butter and bake in a slow oven at 325 for about an hour.

Serve hot.

By Italian standards, the sauce should be homemade, fresh and flavorful, but can be prepared with the simplest of ingredients, such as olive oil, butter, onion, garlic and herbs.

HEMP AND CHIA SEED OATMEAL

Ingredients
- 12 cup quick cook oats gluten-free (or steel cut)
- 1 cup water
- pink Himalayan salt dash of
- 1 tablespoon flax meal
- 3 tablespoons hemp seeds

- 1 tablespoon chia seeds
- 1-2 tablespoons maple syrup
- 14 cup almond milk or less
- fresh berries and fruit
- chopped nuts or seeds optional
- 1 tablespoon almond butter optional

Direction

Rinse and chop any fresh fruit. Set aside.

Stove Top

Boil water and add the oats. Cook about 1 minute over medium heat, stirring occasionally.

Microwave

Combine water and oats in a medium microwaveable bowl. Microwave 1 12 to 2 minutes.

Add The Oatmeal Extras

Add flax meal, chia seeds, hemp seeds, maple syrup, a dash of salt and up to 14 cup almond milk (depending how "soup-like" you like it). Mix well.

Top with favorite toppings such as fresh fruit, nuts, and almond butter.

CAPRESE SALAD SKEWERS

INGREDIENTS
- 1 pint cherry tomatoes, rinsed and dried
- Extra-virgin olive oil

- Flaky sea salt
- 8 ounces bocconcini
- Small leaves from about 12 a bunch of basil, rinsed and dried

Directions

Add the cherry tomatoes to a medium mixing bowl, drizzle with olive oil, sprinkle generously with salt, and gently toss to coat.

Add the bocconcini to a second medium mixing bowl, drizzle with olive oil, sprinkle generously with salt, and gently to toss to coat.

Thread the tomatoes, bocconcini, and basil onto the skewers in this order: tomato, basil (fold larger leaves in half), bocconcini, tomato, basil, bocconcini. Repeat with the remaining skewers. Arrange on a platter.

EASY LEMON BUTTER BAKED FISH

INGREDIENTS
- 800 g1,7lbs White fish, boned (Approximately 200g7oz per person)
- 3 tbsp butter
- 4 garlic cloves crushed
- 3 tbsp fresh lemon juice
- 2 tsp dried oreganothyme
- salt and pepper to taste
- asparagus washed and trimmed

Direction

Pre-heat the oven to 200ºC400ºF and line a sheet pan with parchmentbaking paper.

Combine the butter, lemon, garlic and herbs in a saucepan and bring to a simmer. Cook for 2-3 minutes until fragrant then remove from the heat and set aside to cool slightly.

Place the fish and asparagus onto the lined sheet pan then season with salt and pepper.

Pour the lemon butter sauce over the fish and asparagus and top the fish with lemon slices (optional).

Place in the oven and bake for 10-12 minutes or until the fish and asparagus are cooked. Fish is cooked when it flakes easily and the flesh is opaque, white throughout.

Remove from the oven and serve.

Mediterranean Diet (1 week) Meal Plan for Beginners

Unlike conventional diets, the Mediterranean diet doesn't restrict you to a daily allotment of calories, fat, or sodium. Instead, it's about what you're eating, from heart-healthy unsaturated fats to satiating, high-fiber foods. Taking these ideals to heart, we've constructed a Mediterranean diet meal plan for beginners from breakfast to dinner. Our recipes maximize flavor and nutrition to create balanced and colorful plates that marry whole grains with vegetables, lean proteins, and more. On top of all of this deliciously nutritious eating, make sure to work physical activity into your day, especially if you have a desk job.

Day 1

Breakfast

Fig & Ricotta Toast

Ingredients
- 1 slice crusty whole-grain bread (½-inch thick)
- ¼ cup part-skim ricotta cheese
- 1 fresh fig or 2 dried, sliced
- 1 teaspoon sliced almonds, toasted

- 1 teaspoon honey Pinch of flaky sea salt, such as Maldon

Directions

Toast bread. Top with ricotta cheese, figs and almonds. Drizzle with honey and sprinkle with sea salt.

LUNCH

GREEN SALAD WITH PITA BREAD & HUMMUS

Ingredients
- 2 cups mixed salad greens
- ½ cup sliced cucumber
- 2 tablespoons grated carrot
- 1½ teaspoons extra-virgin olive oil
- Pinch of salt
- Pinch of ground pepper
- 1 6½-inch whole-wheat pita bread, toasted
- ¼ cup hummus

Direction

Arrange greens, cucumber and carrot on a large plate. Drizzle with oil and vinegar. Sprinkle with salt and pepper. Serve with pita and hummus

DINNER

Walnut-Rosemary Crusted Salmon

Ingredients
- 2 teaspoons Dijon mustard
- 1 clove garlic, minced
- ¼ teaspoon lemon zest
- 1 teaspoon lemon juice
- 1 teaspoon chopped fresh rosemary
- ½ teaspoon honey
- ½ teaspoon kosher salt
- ¼ teaspoon crushed red pepper
- 3 tablespoons panko breadcrumbs
- 3 tablespoons finely chopped walnuts
- 1 teaspoon extra-virgin olive oil
- 1 (1 pound) skinless salmon fillet, fresh or frozen
- Olive oil cooking spray

Directions

Preheat oven to 425°F. Line a large rimmed baking sheet with parchment paper. Combine mustard, garlic, lemon zest, lemon juice, rosemary, honey, salt and crushed red pepper in a small bowl. Combine panko, walnuts and oil in another small bowl. Place salmon on the prepared baking sheet. Spread the mustard mixture over the fish and sprinkle with the panko mixture, pressing to adhere. Lightly coat with cooking spray. Bake until the fish flakes easily with a fork, about 8 to 12 minutes, depending on thickness.

Day 2

Breakfast

Muesli with Raspberries

Ingredients
- ⅓ cup muesli
- 1 cup raspberries
- ¾ cup low-fat milk

Direction
Top muesli with raspberries and serve with milk.

Lunch

Roasted Veggie & Quinoa Salad

Ingredients
- 2 cups mixed salad greens
- 1 cup roasted root vegetables
- ½ cup cooked quinoa
- 1-2 tablespoons vinaigrette
- 1 tablespoon crumbled feta cheese
- 1 tablespoon sunflower seeds

Direction

Combine greens, roasted vegetables and quinoa; drizzle with vinaigrette. Top the salad with feta and sunflower seeds.

To make ahead: Assemble recipe, cover and store in the refrigerator for up to 1 day. If storing for more than 1 day, refrigerate mixed greens separately and combine with the other ingredients just before serving.

DINNER

TOMATO & ARTICHOKE GNOCCHI

Ingredients

- 2 tablespoons extra-virgin olive oil, divided
- 1 16-ounce package shelf-stable gnocchi
- 1 small onion, sliced
- 1 small red bell pepper, diced
- 4 large cloves garlic, thinly sliced
- 1 tablespoon chopped fresh oregano, plus more for garnish
- 1 15-ounce can chickpeas, rinsed
- 1 14-ounce can no-salt-added diced tomatoes
- 1 9-ounce box frozen artichoke hearts, thawed and chopped
- 8 pitted Kalamata olives, sliced1 tablespoon red-wine vinegar
- ¼ teaspoon ground pepper

Direction

Heat 1 tablespoon oil in a large nonstick skillet over medium-high heat. Add gnocchi and cook, stirring often, until plumped and starting to brown, about 5 minutes. Transfer to a bowl and cover to keep warm. Reduce heat to medium. Add the remaining 1 tablespoon oil and onion to the pan. Cook, stirring occasionally, until starting to brown, 2 to 3 minutes. Add bell pepper; cook, stirring occasionally, until crisp-tender, about 3 minutes. Add garlic and oregano; cook, stirring, for 30 seconds. Add chickpeas, tomatoes and artichokes; cook, stirring, until hot, about 3 minutes. Stir in olives, vinegar, pepper and the gnocchi. Sprinkle with oregano, if desired.

Day 3

Breakfast

Creamy Mediterranean Paninis

Ingredients
- 12 cup panins
- Mayonnaise Dressing with Olive Oil, divided
- 14 cup chopped fresh basil leaves
- 2 tablespoons finely chopped oil-cured black olives
- 8 slices rustic whole grain bread (about 12-inch thick)
- 1 small zucchini, thinly sliced
- 4 slices provolone cheese

- 1 jar (7 oz.) roasted red peppers, drained and sliced

Direction

Combine 14 cup Hellmann's® or Best Foods® Mayonnaise Dressing with Olive Oil, basil with olives in small bowl. Evenly spread bread slices with mayonnaise mixture, then layer 4 bread slices with zucchini, provolone, peppers and bacon. Top with remaining 4 bread slices.

Spread remaining Mayonnaise on outside of sandwiches and cook in 12-inch nonstick skillet or grill pan over medium heat, turning once, until sandwiches are golden brown and cheese is melted, about 4 minutes.

LUNCH

TOMATO & ARTICHOKE GNOCCHI

Ingredients
- 2 tablespoons extra-virgin olive oil, divided
- 1 16-ounce package shelf-stable gnocchi
- 1 small onion, sliced
- 1 small red bell pepper, diced
- 4 large cloves garlic, thinly sliced

- 1 tablespoon chopped fresh oregano, plus more for garnish
- 1 15-ounce can chickpeas, rinsed
- 1 14-ounce can no-salt-added diced tomatoes
- 1 9-ounce box frozen artichoke hearts, thawed and chopped
- 8 pitted Kalamata olives, sliced
- 1 tablespoon red-wine vinegar
- ¼ teaspoon ground pepper

Direction

Heat 1 tablespoon oil in a large nonstick skillet over medium-high heat. Add gnocchi and cook, stirring often, until plumped and starting to brown, about 5 minutes. Transfer to a bowl and cover to keep warm. Reduce heat to medium. Add the remaining 1 tablespoon oil and onion to the pan. Cook, stirring occasionally, until starting to brown, 2 to 3 minutes. Add bell pepper; cook, stirring occasionally, until crisp-tender, about 3 minutes. Add garlic and oregano; cook, stirring, for 30 seconds. Add chickpeas, tomatoes and artichokes; cook, stirring, until hot, about 3 minutes. Stir in olives, vinegar, pepper and the gnocchi. Sprinkle with oregano, if desired.

DINNER

COD IN TOMATO CREAM SAUCE

Ingredients

- 1-1¼ pounds cod or tilapia fillets, cut into 4 pieces
- 3 teaspoons chopped fresh thyme, divided
- ½ teaspoon salt, divided
- ¼ teaspoon freshly ground pepper
- 1 tablespoon extra-virgin olive oil
- 1 shallot, chopped
- 2 cloves garlic, minced¾ cup white wine
- 1 14-ounce can diced tomatoes
- ¼ cup heavy cream or half-and-half
- ½ teaspoon cornstarch

Direction

Season fish with 1 teaspoon thyme, ¼ teaspoon salt and pepper. Heat oil in a large skillet over medium heat. Add shallot, garlic and 1 teaspoon thyme; cook, stirring, until beginning to soften, about 1 minute. Add wine, tomatoes and the fish to the pan; bring to a simmer. Cover and cook until the fish is cooked through, 4 to 6 minutes. Transfer the fish to a large plate; keep warm. Whisk cream and cornstarch in a small bowl. Add to the pan, along with the remaining 1 teaspoon thyme and ¼ teaspoon salt. Cook, stirring, for 1 minute. Divide the fish and sauce among 4 shallow bowls

DAY 4

BREAKFAST

CREAMY BLUEBERRY-PECAN OVERNIGHT OATS

Ingredients
- ½ cup old-fashioned rolled oats
- ½ cup water
- Pinch of salt
- ½ cup blueberries, fresh or frozen, thawed
- 2 tablespoons nonfat plain Greek yogurt
- 1 tablespoon toasted chopped pecans
- 2 teaspoons pure maple syrup

Direction

Combine oats, water and salt in a jar or bowl. Cover and refrigerate overnight. In the morning, heat if desired, and top with blueberries, yogurt, pecans and syrup.

LUNCH

ROASTED VEGGIE & HUMMUS PITA POCKETS

Ingredients
- 1 6½- inch whole-wheat pita bread
- 4 tablespoons hummus
- ½ cup mixed salad greens

- ½ cup Sheet-Pan Roasted Root Vegetables, roughly chopped
- 1 tablespoon crumbled feta cheese

Direction

Cut pita bread in half. Spread 2 tablespoons hummus inside each half of the pita pocket. Stuff each pita pocket with greens, roasted vegetables and feta.

Dinner

Chicken & White Bean Soup

Ingredients
- 2 teaspoons extra-virgin olive oil
- 2 leeks, white and light green parts only, cut into ¼-inch rounds
- 1 tablespoon chopped fresh sage, or ¼ teaspoon dried
- 2 14-ounce cans reduced-sodium chicken broth
- 2 cups water
- 1 15-ounce can cannellini beans, rinsed
- 1 2-pound roasted chicken, skin discarded, meat removed from bones and shredded

Direction

Heat oil in a Dutch oven over medium-high heat. Add leeks and cook, stirring often, until soft, about 3 minutes. Stir in sage and continue cooking until aromatic, about 30 seconds. Stir in broth and water, increase heat to high, cover and bring to a boil. Add beans and chicken and cook, uncovered, stirring occasionally, until heated through, about 3 minutes. Serve hot.

Day 5

Breakfast

Muesli with Raspberries

Ingredients
- ⅓ cup muesli
- 1 cup raspberries
- ¾ cup low-fat milk

Direction
Top muesli with raspberries and serve with milk.

Lunch

Chicken & White Bean Soup

Ingredients
- 2 teaspoons extra-virgin olive oil
- 2 leeks, white and light green parts only, cut into ¼-inch rounds

- 1 tablespoon chopped fresh sage, or ¼ teaspoon dried
- 2 14-ounce cans reduced-sodium chicken broth
- 2 cups water
- 1 15-ounce can cannellini beans, rinsed
- 1 2-pound roasted chicken, skin discarded, meat removed from bones and shredded (4 cups)

Directions

Heat oil in a Dutch oven over medium-high heat. Add leeks and cook, stirring often, until soft, about 3 minutes. Stir in sage and continue cooking until aromatic, about 30 seconds. Stir in broth and water, increase heat to high, cover and bring to a boil. Add beans and chicken and cook, uncovered, stirring occasionally, until heated through, about 3 minutes. Serve hot.

DINNER

ROASTED ROOT VEGETABLES WITH GOAT CHEESE

Ingredients
Polenta

- 2 cups low-sodium vegetable or chicken broth
- ½ cup polenta fine cornmeal or corn grits

- ¼ cup goat cheese
- 1 tablespoon extra-virgin olive oil or butter
- ¼ teaspoon kosher salt
- ¼ teaspoon ground pepper

VEGETABLES

- 1 tablespoon extra-virgin olive oil or butter
- 1 clove garlic, smashed
- 2 cups roasted root vegetables
- 1 tablespoon torn fresh sage
- 2 teaspoons prepared pesto
- Fresh parsley for garnish

Direction

To prepare polenta: Bring broth to a boil in a medium saucepan. Reduce heat to low and gradually add polenta (or cornmeal or grits), whisking vigorously to avoid clumping. Cover and cook for 10 minutes. Stir, cover and continue cooking until thickened and creamy, about 10 minutes more. Stir in goat cheese, oil (or butter), salt and pepper. Meanwhile, to prepare vegetables: Heat oil (or butter) in a medium skillet over medium heat. Add garlic and cook, stirring, until fragrant, about 1 minute. Add roasted vegetables and cook, stirring often, until heated through, 2 to 4 minutes. Stir in sage and cook until fragrant, about 1 minute more. Serve the vegetables over the polenta, topped with pesto. Garnish with parsley, if desired.

Day 6

Breakfast

Creamy Blueberry-Pecan Overnight Oats

Ingredients

- ½ cup old-fashioned rolled oats
- ½ cup water
- Pinch of salt
- ½ cup blueberries, fresh or frozen, thawed
- 2 tablespoons nonfat plain Greek yogurt
- 1 tablespoon toasted chopped pecans
- 2 teaspoons pure maple syrup

Directions

Combine oats, water and salt in a jar or bowl. Cover and refrigerate overnight. In the morning, heat if desired, and top with blueberries, yogurt, pecans and syrup.

Lunch

Chickpea & Veggie Grain Bowl

Ingredients

1 cup cooked quinoa

- 1 cup mixed salad greens
- 1 cup roasted root vegetables
- ¼ cup canned chickpeas, rinsed
- 1 tablespoon crumbled feta cheese

Direction
Combine quinoa, greens, roasted vegetables, chickpeas and feta in a bowl.

DINNER

MEDITERRANEAN CHICKEN & ORZO

Ingredients
- 1 pound boneless, skinless chicken breasts, trimmed
- 1 cup low-sodium chicken broth
- 2 medium tomatoes, chopped
- 1 medium onion, halved and sliced
- Zest and juice of 1 lemon
- 1 teaspoon herbes de Provence
- ½ teaspoon salt
- ½ teaspoon ground pepper
- ¾ cup whole-wheat orzo
- ⅓ cup quartered black or green olives
- 2 tablespoons chopped fresh parsley

Direction
Combine quinoa, greens, roasted vegetables, chickpeas and feta in a bowl.

Day 7

Breakfast

Rainbow Frittata

Ingredients
- Nonstick cooking spray
- ¼ cup ½-inch pieces sweet potato
- ¼ cup ½-inch pieces yellow sweet pepper
- ¼ cup coarsely chopped fresh broccoli
- ½ teaspoon snipped fresh thyme
- ⅛ teaspoon salt⅛ teaspoon cracked black pepper
- 1 avocado, halved, seeded, peeled and thinly sliced
- 8 omega-3 enriched eggs
- 1 teaspoon snipped fresh basil
- 5½ cups grape or cherry tomatoes, halved
- Sriracha sauce

Direction
Preheat oven to 350 F. Coat an oven-going 10-inch nonstick skillet with cooking spray. Add sweet potato, sweet pepper and broccoli; cook and stir over medium 5 to 7 minutes or until tender. In a medium bowl whisk

together eggs, basil, thyme, salt and black pepper. Pour mixture over vegetables in skillet. Cook, without stirring, until mixture begins to set on bottom and around edges. Using a spatula, lift egg mixture so uncooked portion flows underneath. Transfer skillet to oven; cook 5 minutes or until egg mixture is set. Remove from oven. Let stand 2 minutes. Top servings with avocado and tomatoes. Drizzle with sriracha.

Lunch

Tuna salad

Ingredients
- 2 cans (6 oz. ea.) tuna, drained and flaked
- 14 cup Mayonnaise Dressing with Olive Oil
- 14 cup chopped pitted ripe olives
- 14 cup drained and chopped roasted red peppers
- 2 green onions, sliced
- 1 tablespoon small capers, rinsed and drained
- 6 slices whole wheat bread

Direction
Combine all ingredients except bread in medium bowl. Arrange, if desired, on greens and serve with bread.

Dinner

Dijon Salmon with Green Bean Pilaf

Ingredients
- 1¼ pounds wild salmon, skinned and cut into 4 portions
- 3 tablespoons extra-virgin olive oil, divided
- 1 tablespoon minced garlic
- ¾ teaspoon salt
- 2 tablespoons mayonnaise
- 2 teaspoons whole-grain mustard
- ½ teaspoon ground pepper, divided
- 12 ounces pretrimmed haricots verts or thin green beans, cut into thirds
- 1 small lemon, zested and cut into 4 wedges
- 2 tablespoons pine nuts
- 1 8-ounce package precooked brown rice
- 2 tablespoons water
- Chopped fresh parsley for garnish

Directions

Preheat oven to 425°F. Line a rimmed baking sheet with foil or parchment paper. Brush salmon with 1 tablespoon oil and place on the prepared baking sheet. Mash garlic and salt into a paste with the side of a chef's knife or a fork. Combine a scant 1 teaspoon of the garlic paste in a small bowl with mayonnaise, mustard and ¼ teaspoon pepper. Spread the mixture on top of the fish. Roast the salmon until it flakes easily with a fork in the thickest part, 6 to 8 minutes per inch of thickness. Meanwhile, heat the remaining 2 tablespoons oil in a large skillet over medium-high heat. Add green beans, lemon zest, pine nuts, the remaining garlic paste and ¼ teaspoon pepper; cook, stirring, until the beans are just tender, 2 to 4 minutes. Reduce heat to medium. Add rice and water and cook, stirring, until hot, 2 to 3 minutes more. Sprinkle the salmon with parsley, if desired, and serve with the green bean pilaf and lemon wedges.

GREAT MEDITERREAN DIET RECIPES

PASTA SALAD

Ingredients
- 8 ounces multigrain farfalle Zest and juice of 1 lemon
- 2 teaspoons olive oil
- 1 13.5- ounce can artichoke hearts packed in water, drained and chopped
- 8 ounces fresh part-skim mozzarella cheese, chopped
- 14 cup chopped bottled roasted red bell pepper
- 14 cup chopped fresh parsley
- 12 cup frozen peas

Direction

Cook pasta according to package instructions, omitting salt and fat.

While pasta cooks, combine zest and juice of 1 lemon and 2 teaspoons olive oil in a large bowl; stir well with a whisk. Add artichoke hearts, cheese, bell pepper, and parsley; toss to combine.

Place peas in a colander; when pasta is cooked, drain pasta over peas. Shake well to drain, but do not run under cold water. Add pasta and peas to artichoke mixture, and toss well until thoroughly combined. Serve warm or at room temperature.

SEAFOOD GRILL WITH SKORDALIA

Ingredients
- 1 pound russet or Yukon gold potatoes
- 8 garlic cloves, peeled
- 1 slice sourdough bread, crust removed
- 14 cup plain Greek low-fat yogurt
- 3 tablespoons olive oil, divided
- Zest and juice of 1 lemon
- 12 teaspoon salt, divided
- 14 teaspoon dried thyme
- 1 pound halibut fillets, cut into 4 pieces
- 2 red bell peppers, quartered
- 1 pound small zucchini, diagonally cut into 1-inch pieces
- 12 red onion, sliced

Direction

Peel potatoes, and chop into 1-inch pieces. Place in a large saucepan, and cover with cold water. Add garlic, and cook over high heat about 15 minutes or until potatoes are easily pierced with a fork.

While potatoes cook, tear bread into 3 or 4 pieces and place in a large bowl. Spoon 2 to 3 tablespoons cooking liquid from potatoes over bread. Stir with a fork until smooth. Add yogurt, 2 tablespoons olive oil, and zest and juice of 1 lemon; stir until a smooth paste forms.

When the potatoes are done, place a large bowl in the sink and set a colander on top. Drain potatoes and garlic, reserving cooking liquid. Transfer potatoes to bread mixture and mash until smooth (a potato ricer works well for this task). Add reserved cooking liquid 2 tablespoons at a time until mixture takes on the consistency of loose mashed potatoes. Stir in ½ teaspoon salt and 2 teaspoons olive oil. Cover and keep warm until ready to serve.

Preheat grill pan over medium-high heat. Drizzle fish with ½ teaspoon olive oil and season with remaining ½ teaspoon salt and thyme. Cook fish 2 to 3 minutes on each side until fish flakes when tested with a fork or until desired degree of doneness. Transfer to a plate; cover and keep warm until ready to serve.

Place bell pepper, zucchini, and red onion in a large bowl. Drizzle with remaining ½ teaspoon olive oil; toss to coat. Arrange bell pepper in grill pan and cook 5 minutes over medium heat. Add zucchini and onion;

cook 10 minutes or until vegetables are tender, turning as necessary to ensure even cooking.

CHICKPEA PATTIES

Ingredients
- 1 (15.5-ounce) can chickpeas, rinsed and drained
- 12 cup fresh flat-leaf parsley
- 1 garlic clove, chopped
- 14 teaspoon ground cumin
- 12 teaspoon kosher salt, divided
- 12 teaspoon black pepper, divided
- 1 egg, whisked
- 4 tablespoons all-purpose flour, divided
- 2 tablespoons olive oil
- 12 cup low-fat Greek-style yogurt
- 3 tablespoons fresh lemon juice
- 8 cups mixed salad greens
- 1 cup grape tomatoes, halved
- 12 small red onion, thinly sliced
- Pita chips (optional)

Direction

Pulse first 4 ingredients (through cumin) and 14 teaspoon each salt and pepper in a food processor until coarsely chopped and mixture comes together. Transfer to a bowl, add egg and 2 tablespoons flour; form into 8 (12-inch-thick) patties. Place remaining flour in a small dish and roll patties in it with floured hands; tap off excess flour.

Heat oil in a nonstick skillet over medium-high heat. Cook patties for 2-3 minutes per side or until golden.

Whisk together the yogurt, lemon juice, and remaining salt and pepper. Divide greens, tomatoes, onion, and patties evenly among 4 plates; drizzle each salad with 2 tablespoons dressing. Serve with pita chips, if desired.

Salmon

Ingredients
- 14 teaspoon salt
- 14 teaspoon black pepper
- 4 (6-ounce) skinless salmon fillets (about 1 inch thick)

Cooking spray

- 2 cups cherry tomatoes, halved
- 12 cup finely chopped zucchini
- 2 tablespoons capers, undrained
- 1 tablespoon olive oil
- 1 (2 14-ounce) can sliced ripe olives, drained

Direction
Preheat oven to 425°.

Sprinkle salt and pepper over both sides of fish. Place fish in a single layer in an 11- x 7-inch baking dish coated with cooking spray. Combine tomatoes and remaining ingredients in a bowl; spoon mixture over fish. Bake at 425° for 22 minutes.

SHRIMP AND PASTA

Ingredients
- 2 teaspoons olive oil Cooking spray
- 2 garlic cloves, minced
- 1 pound medium shrimp, peeled and deveined
- 2 cups chopped plum tomato
- 14 cup thinly sliced fresh basil
- 13 cup chopped pitted kalamata olives
- 2 tablespoons capers, drained
- 14 teaspoon freshly ground black pepper
- 4 cups hot cooked angel hair pasta (about 8 ounces uncooked pasta)
- 14 cup (2 ounces) crumbled feta cheese

Direction

Heat olive oil in a large nonstick skillet coated with cooking spray over medium-high heat. Add garlic; sauté 30 seconds. Add shrimp; sauté 1 minute. Add tomato and basil; reduce heat, and simmer 3 minutes or until tomato is tender. Stir in kalamata olives, capers, and black pepper.

Combine shrimp mixture and pasta in a large bowl; toss well. Top with cheese.

Portobello Mushrooms with Mediterranean Stuffing

Ingredients
- 4 (4-inch) portobello caps (about 34 pound)
- 14 cup finely chopped onion
- 14 cup finely chopped celery
- 14 cup finely chopped carrot
- 14 cup finely chopped red bell pepper
- 14 cup finely chopped green bell pepper
- 14 teaspoon dried Italian seasoning
- 2 garlic cloves, minced Cooking spray
- 3 cups (14-inch) cubed French bread, toasted
- 12 cup vegetable broth
- 12 cup (2 ounces) feta cheese, crumbled
- 3 tablespoons low-fat balsamic vinaigrette, divided
- 4 teaspoons grated fresh Parmesan cheese
- 14 teaspoon black pepper
- 4 cups mixed salad greens

Directions

Preheat oven to 350°.

Remove stems from mushrooms, and finely chop stems to measure 14 cup. Discard remaining stems.

Heat a large nonstick skillet over medium heat; coat pan with cooking spray. Add onion mixture to pan; cook 10 minutes or until vegetables are tender. Combine onion mixture and bread in a large bowl, tossing to combine. Slowly add broth to bread mixture, tossing to coat. Add feta; toss gently.

Remove brown gills from the undersides of mushroom caps using a spoon; discard gills. Place mushrooms, stem side up, on a baking sheet coated with cooking spray. Brush mushrooms evenly with 1 tablespoon vinaigrette. Sprinkle Parmesan and black pepper evenly over mushrooms; top each with 12 cup bread mixture. Bake at 350° for 25 minutes or until mushrooms are tender.

Combine remaining 2 tablespoons vinaigrette and greens, tossing gently. Place 1 cup greens on each of 4 plates; top each serving with 1 mushroom.

GREEK-STYLE PICNIC SALAD

Ingredients
- 2 cups uncooked white rice
- 1 cup boiling water
- 34 cup sun-dried tomatoes, packed without oil
- 1 12 tablespoons olive oil, divided

- 8 cups bagged prewashed spinach (about 8 ounces)
- 2 garlic cloves, minced
- 2 cups (8 ounces) reduced-fat feta cheese, crumbled
- 14 cup chopped pitted kalamata olives
- 1 teaspoon dried oregano
- 12 teaspoon salt
- 12 teaspoon freshly ground black pepper
- 1 (15 12-ounce) can chickpeas (garbanzo beans), rinsed and drained
- 3 tablespoons pine nuts, toasted
- 10 lemon wedges (optional)

Direction

Cook rice according to package directions, omitting salt and fat. Cool to room temperature; set aside.

Combine boiling water and sun-dried tomatoes in a bowl; let stand 30 minutes or until soft. Drain and cut into 1-inch pieces.

Heat 1 12 teaspoons oil in a large skillet over medium-high heat. Add spinach and garlic; sauté 3 minutes or until spinach wilts. Combine rice, tomatoes, spinach mixture, cheese, and next 5 ingredients (through chickpeas). Drizzle with remaining 1 tablespoon oil; toss gently to coat. Sprinkle with nuts; serve with lemon wedges, if desired.

STUFFED TOMATOES

Ingredients
- 2 large tomatoes
- 12 cup packaged garlic croutons
- 14 cup (1 ounce) crumbled goat cheese
- 14 cup sliced pitted kalamata olives
- 2 tablespoons reduced-fat vinaigrette or Italian salad dressing
- 2 tablespoons chopped fresh thyme or basil

Direction
Preheat broiler.

Cut tomatoes in half crosswise. Use your finger to push out and discard seeds; use a paring knife to cut out the pulp, leaving 2 shells. Chop pulp, and transfer to a medium bowl. Place hollowed tomatoes, cut sides down, on a paper towel; drain 5 minutes. Add croutons, goat cheese, olives, dressing, and thyme or basil to pulp; mix well. Mound mixture into hollowed tomatoes.

Place tomatoes on a baking sheet or broiler pan. Broil 4-5 inches from heat until hot and cheese melts (about 5 minutes). Serve immediately.

BREAKFAST COUSCOUS

Ingredients
- 3 cups 1% low-fat milk
- 1 (2-inch) cinnamon stick

- 1 cup uncooked whole-wheat couscous
- 12 cup chopped dried apricots
- 14 cup dried currants
- 6 teaspoons dark brown sugar, divided
- 14 teaspoon salt
- 4 teaspoons butter, melted and divided

Direction

Combine milk and cinnamon stick in a large saucepan over medium-high heat; heat 3 minutes or until small bubbles form around inner edge of pot (about 180°). Do not boil.

Remove from heat; stir in couscous, apricots, currants, 4 teaspoons brown sugar, and salt. Cover the mixture, and let it stand 15 minutes. Remove and discard cinnamon stick. Divide couscous among each of 4 bowls, and top each with 1 teaspoon melted butter and 12 teaspoon brown sugar. Serve immediately.

Pizza

Ingredients
- 1 (12-inch) prepared pizza crust
- 14 teaspoon crushed red pepper
- 14 teaspoon dried Italian seasoning
- 1 cup (4 ounces) crumbled goat cheese
- 3 sliced plum tomatoes (14-inch-thick slices)
- 6 chopped pitted kalamata olives

- 1 (14-ounce) can quartered artichoke hearts, drained Cooking spray
- 14 cup chopped fresh basil or 4 teaspoons dried basil

Direction

Preheat oven to 450°.

Sprinkle the pizza crust with crushed red pepper and dried Italian seasoning.

Sprinkle the crumbled goat cheese evenly on the crust, leaving a 12-inch border. Using the back of a spoon, gently press the cheese down on the pizza crust.

Arrange the plum tomato slices, chopped olives, and quartered artichoke hearts on the pizza as desired.

Place the pizza on a baking sheet coated with cooking spray, and bake 10-12 minutes or until the crust is crisp and the cheese is bubbly. Sprinkle the chopped basil over the top and serve hot.

GRILLED VEGETABLE TAGINE

Ingredients
- 1 small red onion
- 2 red bell peppers, quartered
- 1 green bell pepper, quartered
- 2 teaspoons balsamic vinegar
- 12 teaspoon kosher salt, divided
- 1 teaspoon olive oil, divided

- 1 34 cups chopped onion
- 2 garlic cloves, minced
- 1 teaspoon ground cumin
- 12 teaspoon fennel seeds, crushed
- 14 teaspoon ground cinnamon
- 1 14 cups water, divided
- 14 cup sliced pitted green olives
- 14 cup golden raisins
- 14 teaspoon freshly ground black pepper
- 1 (28-ounce) can diced tomatoes, undrained
- 6 small red potatoes, quartered Cooking spray
- 23 cup uncooked couscous
- 14 cup pine nuts, toasted

Direction

put red onion into 4 wedges, leaving root end intact. Place red onion, bell peppers, vinegar, 14 teaspoon salt, and 12 teaspoon oil in a zip-top plastic bag. Seal bag; toss well to coat.

Prepare grill.

Heat 12 teaspoon oil in a large nonstick skillet over medium-high heat. Add chopped onion and garlic; sauté 3 minutes. Add cumin, fennel, and cinnamon; sauté 1 minute. Add 14 teaspoon salt, 14 cup water, olives, raisins, black pepper, tomatoes, and potatoes; bring to a boil. Cover, reduce heat, and simmer 25 minutes or until potatoes are just tender.

Remove bell peppers and red onion from bag, discarding marinade; place on grill rack coated with cooking spray. Grill 10 minutes, turning frequently.

Bring 1 cup of water to a boil in a medium saucepan; gradually stir in couscous. Remove from heat; cover and let stand 5 minutes. Fluff with a fork. Serve tomato mixture over couscous. Top with grilled bell peppers and red onions; sprinkle with pine nuts.

GREEK SALMON BURGERS

Ingredients
- 1 pound skinless salmon fillets, cut into 2-inch pieces
- 12 cup panko
- 1 large egg white
- 1 pinch kosher salt
- 14 teaspoon freshly ground black pepper
- 12 cup cucumber slices
- 14 cup crumbled feta cheese
- 4 (2.5-oz) ciabatta rolls, toasted

Directions

In the bowl of a food processor, pulse salmon, panko, and egg white until salmon is finely chopped.

Form salmon into 4 (4-inch) patties; season with salt and pepper.

Heat grill to medium-high; cook, turning once, until burgers are just cooked through (5-7 minutes per side). Serve with desired toppings and buns.

STUFFED ROASTED RED PEPPERS

Ingredients
- 6 large red bell peppers
- 1 tablespoon olive oil
- 4 garlic cloves, minced
- 6 ounces fresh spinach
- 1 tablespoon fresh lemon juice
- 1 teaspoon salt
- 34 cup uncooked couscous (about 2 cups cooked)
- 12 cup crumbled feta cheese

Direction

Roast the bell peppers on a gas stove's open flame, turning them with tongs, until the skins are blackened, for about 2-3 minutes; or roast them on a rack under the broiler 2 inches from the heat, turning them every 5 minutes, for about 15 minutes. Transfer peppers to a bowl, cover with plastic wrap, and let them cool. When cool enough to handle, peel peppers starting at the stem end, carefully cut off the tops with a paring knife, and rinse out any seeds. Set aside.

Lightly coat a sauté pan with olive oil; place over medium heat. Sauté garlic until it begins to turn golden, about 1 minute. Add spinach; cook over medium heat until it wilts, about 2 minutes. Remove pan from heat. Stir in lemon juice and salt; place spinach in a bowl. Preheat oven to 350°.

In a small pot, cook couscous according to package directions (about 5 minutes). Using a spatula, add the couscous and the feta cheese to the wilted spinach, and mix well.

Line a baking sheet with aluminum foil. Generously stuff all the peppers with couscous-spinach stuffing, and place on a baking sheet. Bake on the center rack for about 8 minutes. Serve immediately.

CHICKEN-GARBANZO SALAD

Ingredients
- 1 (9-ounce) package frozen cooked chopped chicken breast, thawed
- 1 (15-ounce) can chickpeas (garbanzo beans), rinsed and drained
- 1 cup chopped seeded cucumber (about 1 small)
- 12 cup chopped green onions (about 4 small)
- 14 cup chopped fresh mint or basil
- 12 cup plain fat-free yogurt
- 2 garlic cloves, minced
- 14 teaspoon salt
- 2 cups prepackaged baby spinach leaves
- 13 cup (1.3 ounces) feta cheese with cracked pepper, crumbled
- 4 lemon wedges

Direction

Combine first 8 ingredients; toss gently. Gently fold in spinach leaves and feta cheese. Serve salad with lemon wedges.

TWO-BEAN GREEK SALAD

Ingredients
- 2 tablespoons red wine vinegar
- 2 teaspoons Dijon mustard
- 3 teaspoons chopped fresh oregano, divided
- 4 1⁄2 teaspoons olive oil, divided
- 1⁄2 teaspoon freshly ground black pepper, divided
- 1 (10-ounce) bag shelled frozen edamame or lima beans
- 3⁄4 pound string beans
- 1 cup grape tomatoes, halved
- 1⁄4 cup pitted kalamata olives, halved
- 2 multigrain pitas, halved horizontally
- 3 ounces haloumi cheese (or ricotta salata), sliced into 4 pieces

Direction

In a serving bowl, whisk together red wine vinegar, Dijon mustard, 2 1⁄2 teaspoons oregano, 2 teaspoons olive oil, and 1⁄4 teaspoon pepper; set aside.

Place steamer basket in saucepan filled with a few inches of water; cook edamame, covered, until tender (about 3 minutes). Transfer edamame to a bowl. Add string beans to steamer; cook, covered, until tender (about 2 minutes). Add beans to edamame. Add tomatoes and olives; toss to combine.

Heat a lightly oiled grill pan over medium-high heat. Brush 1 teaspoon oil on one side of pitas; grill, turning, until golden (about 2 minutes). Transfer pitas to a plate. Brush 12 teaspoon oil evenly on one side of cheese slices; sprinkle with the remaining oregano and pepper. Grill cheese, seasoned side down, until marks form (about 1 minute); transfer to a plate.

Place 1 pita half on each of 4 plates; top with bean salad and cheese. Drizzle with remaining olive oil.

Mediterranean Bowl with greens

Ingredients
FALAFEL

- 12 batch Classic Vegan Falafel PARSLEY SALAD
- 2 cups fresh chopped parsley
- 12 cup diced tomato
- 14 cup diced red onion
- 2 Tbsp lemon juice
- 1 pinch sea salt
- 1 Tbsp extra virgin (or regular) olive oil (optional)

SAUCES

- Tahini Sauce
- Chili Garlic Sauce
- Garlic Dill Sauce

FOR SERVING

- Hummus
- optional: Mixed greens
- Kalamata or green olives, pitted
- Pita Pita chips Flatbread

Direction

First prepare falafel by following this recipe. You will only need 12 falafel, which is about half of the recipe. I like to make a batch ahead of time and keep them uncooked in my freezer so I just have to slightly thaw and pan-fry them when I want a Mediterranean Bowl! This keeps prepcook time under 30 minutes.

Prepare the parsley salad by adding parsley, tomato, onion, lemon juice, salt and olive oil (optional) to a medium mixing bowl and tossing to combine. Set aside.

To serve, divide salad greens and parsley salad between two serving bowls and top with hummus, olives, 6 falafel each and tahini sauce. I also prefer some fresh lemon juice and chili garlic sauce.

Best when fresh!

POTATO HASH WITH ASPARAGUS, CHICKPEAS AND POACHED EGGS

INGREDIENTS

- Private Reserve extra virgin olive oil
- 1 small yellow onion, chopped
- 2 garlic cloves, chopped
- 2 russet potatoes, diced
- Salt and pepper
- 1 cup canned chickpeas, drained and rinsed
- 1 lb baby asparagus, hard ends removed, chopped into 14 inch pieces
- 1 12 tsp ground allspice
- 1 tsp Za'atar
- 1 tsp dried oregano
- 1 tsp sweet paprika or smoked paprika
- 1 tsp coriander
- Pinch sugar
- 4 eggs (to be poached)
- Water
- 1 tsp White Vinegar
- 1 small red onion, finely chopped
- 2 Roma tomatoes, chopped
- 12 cup crumbled feta
- 1 cup chopped fresh parsley, stems removed

Direction

Heat 1 12 tbsp olive oil in a large cast-iron skillet. Turn the heat to medium-high and add the chopped onions, garlic and potatoes. Season with salt and pepper. Cook for 5-7 minutes, stirring frequently until the potatoes are tender (some of the potatoes may gain a bit of a golden crust, which is good!)

Add the chickpeas, asparagus, a dash more salt and pepper and the spices. Stir to combine. Cook for another 5-7 minutes. Turn the heat to low to keep the potato hash warm; stir regularly.

Meanwhile, bring a medium pot of water to a steady simmer and add 1 tsp vinegar. Break the eggs into a bowl. Stir the simmering water gently and carefully slide the eggs in. The egg whites should warp around the yoke. Cook for 3 minutes exactly, then remove the eggs from the simmering water and onto kitchen towel to drain briefly. Season with salt and pepper.

Remove the potato hash from the heat and add the chopped red onions, tomatoes, feta and parsley. Top with the poached eggs. Enjoy!

ISRAELI PASTA SALAD

Ingredients
- 12 pound small bow tie or other small pasta
- 13 cup cucumber, finely diced (I like to use small Persian cucumbers)
- 13 cup radish, finely diced
- 13 cup tomato, finely diced (drain excess liquid)
- 13 cup yellow bell pepper, finely diced
- 13 cup orange bell pepper, finely diced
- 13 cup black olives, finely diced
- 13 cup green olives, halved
- 13 cup red onion, finely diced

- 13 cup pepperoncini, diced
- 13 cup feta cheese, finely diced
- lots of fresh thyme leaves
- 1 tsp dried oregano
- salt and fresh cracked black pepper to taste

dressing

- 14 cup, plus more, olive oil
- juice of 1 lemon

direction

Cook the pasta in well salted water until just al dente, don't over cook. I usually cook it at least 2 minutes under the time listed on the package. Drain and rinse in cold water.

Put the well drained (not dripping wet) pasta in a bowl and toss with a little olive oil so it doesn't stick together. Add the veggies, oregano, thyme, and salt and pepper. Hold out the feta cheese until the end.

Add the 14 cup olive oil and lemon juice and toss well. Gently fold in the feta cheese.

Refrigerate the salad for at least 2 hours, up to overnight. Taste before serving, you may want to add more olive oil, lemon, salt, or pepper.

Garnish with fresh thyme.

Cauliflower Pizza with Greek Yogurt Pesto & Grilled

Ingredients
For the cauliflower crust:

- 12 Cups Cauliflower cut into florets (about 2 medium heads or 3 lbs)
- 1 Tbsp + 1 tsp Garlic minced
- 12 tsp Salt
- 1 tsp Italian Seasoning
- Pepper
- 1 13 Cup + 4 Tbsp Parmesan cheese grated and divided (about 3.5 oz)
- 2 Large egg whites
- For the Greek yogurt basil sauce:
- 12 Cup Plain Non-fat Greek yogurt
- 12 Cup firmly packed Fresh basil roughly chopped
- 2 tsp Garlic minced
- 1 Tbsp Olive oil
- Saltpepper to taste

For topping:

- 1 Small zucchini sliced
- 3 inch Roma Tomatoes sliced 12 thick *
- 12 Tbsp Olive oil
- 12 Cup Parmesan Cheese grated
- Fresh basil for garnish

Direction

Preheat your oven to 400 degrees and line a pizza pan with parchment paper.

In a large food processor, process the cauliflower into it is fine, and the texture of rice. I did mine in 4 batches.

Place the cauliflower into a LARGE bowl and microwave for 7 minutes, stir, and microwave for an additional 7 minutes. Then, let the cauliflower stand until cool enough to handle, 10-15 minutes.

Dump the cauliflower into a thin kitchen towel ** (I did mine into two batches) and ring out ALL the excess moisture. Put some muscle into it and really get out as much as you can, as this is the key to a not-soggy crust.

Transfer the cauliflower back into a large bowl and add in the garlic, salt, Italian season, a pinch of pepper and 1 13 cups of the Parmesan. Stir until well combined and then add the egg whites, mixing until well combined.

Divide the cauliflower into 4 balls (about a heaping 12 cup each) and spread onto on the pizza pan, leaving a ridge for the crust.

Bake until golden brown, about 30 minutes.

While the pizza bakes, Combine the Greek yogurt, basil and garlic in a small food processor (mine is 3 cups) until smooth and creamy, scraping the sides down as necessary.

With the food processor on, stream in the olive oil until well mixed. Set aside.

Then, preheat your grill to medium-high heat.

Combine the sliced zucchini, tomato and olive oil in a small bowl and season with a pinch of salt and pepper. Grill until charred, about 2-3 minutes a side. Place onto a plate and set aside. Keep your grill on.

Once the pizza is cooked, remove them from the oven and preheat your broiler to high heat for 3 minutes. Take the remaining 4 Tbsp of cheese and sprinkle it onto the pizzas (1 Tbsp each) and broil for 2-3 minutes until golden brown and melted.

Spread some of the Greek yogurt sauce on each pizza and then top with the grilled veggies and sprinkle with remaining cheese.

Place the pizzas onto the grill just until the cheese melts, about 2-3 minutes.

DEVOUR immediately.

GREEK FARRO SALAD

INGREDIENTS:

FOR THE SALAD:

- 1 tablespoon olive oil
- 1 ½ cups pearled farro*
- 1 ¼ cups water
- 2 ½ cups low-sodium vegetable broth
- 2 cups roughly chopped baby spinach leaves
- ½ small red onion, thinly sliced

- 1 cucumber, peeled and chopped
- 1 small green pepper, chopped
- 1 pint cherry tomatoes, halved
- ¾ cup crumbled feta
- 1 can chickpeas, drained and rinsed

FOR THE DRESSING:

- 2 tablespoons freshly squeezed lemon juice
- 1 tablespoon red wine vinegar
- 1 tablespoon honey
- ¼ teaspoon oregano
- ¼ teaspoon salt
- pinch of red pepper flakes
- ¼ cup olive oil

Direction

To make the salad – set a medium saucepan over medium heat. Add in the olive oil. When hot, add in the farro and cook for 1 minute, stirring frequently. Add in the water and broth. Turn up the heat and bring to a boil. Cover, reduce the heat to medium-low and let simmer for about 30 to 35 minutes, until the farro is tender but still slightly chewy. Drain off any excess liquid (if there is any) and then transfer to a large bowl.

Immediately add the spinach to the bowl and toss to combine, so the heat will wilt the spinach a bit. Let cool for about 15 to 20 minutes.

Add in the red onion, cucumber, pepper, tomatoes, feta and chickpeas. Toss to combine.

To make the dressing – add the lemon juice, vinegar, honey, oregano, salt and red pepper to a small bowl. Whisk to combine. Add in the olive oil and whisk vigorously until smooth. Start by pouring some of the dressing into the bowl with the farro. Toss to combine and then taste. Slowly add in more of the dressing to your taste (I usually add all of it). Season with additional salt red pepper if needed. Serve at room temperature or cold

ONE POT GREEK CHICKEN & LEMON RICE

Ingredients
- CHICKEN AND MARINADE
- 5 chicken thighs, skin on, bone in (about 1 kg 2 lb)(Note 1)
- 1 - 2 lemons, use the zest + 4 tbsp lemon juice (Note 7)
- 1 tbsp dried oregano
- 4 garlic cloves, minced
- 12 tsp salt
- RICE
- 1 12 tbsp olive oil, separated
- 1 small onion, finely diced
- 1 cup 180g long grain rice (Note 6 for other rice)
- 1 12 cups 375 ml chicken broth stock
- 34 cup 185ml water
- 1 tbsp dried oregano
- 34 tsp salt
- Black pepper

GARNISH

- Finely chopped parsley or oregano (optional)
- Fresh lemon zest (highly recommended)

Direction

Combine the Chicken and Marinade ingredients in a ziplock bag and set aside for at least 20 minutes but preferably overnight.

TO COOK

Preheat oven to 180C350F.

Remove chicken from marinade, but reserve the Marinade.

Heat 12 tbsp olive oil in a deep, heavy based skillet (Note 2) over medium high heat.

Place the chicken in the skillet, skin side down, and cook until golden brown, then turn and cook the other side until golden brown. Remove the chicken and set aside.

Pour off fat and wipe the pan with a scrunched up ball of paper towel (to remove black bits), then return to the stove.

Heat 1 tbsp olive oil in the skillet over medium high heat. Add the onion and sauté for a few minutes until translucent. Then add the remaining Rice ingredients and reserved Marinade.

Let the liquid come to a simmer and let it simmer for 30 seconds. Place the chicken on top then place a lid on the skillet (Note 3). Bake in the oven for 35 minutes.

Then remove the lid and bake for a further 10 minutes, or until all the liquid is absorbed and the rice is tender (so 45 minutes in total).

Remove from the oven and allow to rest for 5 to 10 minutes before serving, garnished with parsley or oregano and fresh lemon zest, if desired

Greek turkey meatball gyro with tzatziki

Ingredients
Turkey Meatball:

- 1 lb. ground turkey
- 14 cup finely diced red onion
- 2 garlic cloves, minced
- 1 teaspoon oregano
- 1 cup chopped fresh spinach
- salt & pepper to season
- 2 tablespoons olive oil
- Tzatziki Sauce:
- 12 cup plain greek yogurt
- 14 cup grated cucumber
- 2 tablespoons lemon juice
- 12 teaspoon dry dill
- 12 teaspoon garlic powder
- salt to taste
- 12 cup thinly sliced red onion
- 1 cup diced tomato
- 1 cup diced cucumber
- 4 whole wheat flatbreads

Direction

To a large bowl add, ground turkey, diced red onion, minced garlic, oregano, fresh spinach, salt, and pepper. Using your hands mix all the ingredients together until meat forms a ball and sticks together.

Then using your hands, form meat mixture into 1" balls. (you should be able to get about 12 meatballs).

Heat a large skillet to medium high heat. Add olive oil to the pan, and then add the meatballs. Cook each side for 3-4 minutes until they are browned on all sides. Remove from the pan and let rest.

In the meantime, to a small bowl add greek yogurt, grated cucumber, lemon juice, dill, garlic powder, and salt to taste. Mix together until everything is combined.

Assemble the gyros: to a flatbread (I like to warm mine up so they are more pliable) add 3 meatballs, sliced red onion, tomato, and cucumber. Then top with Tzatziki sauce.

SPINACH, FETA & ARTICHOKE MATZO MINA

Ingredients
- 6 sheets matzo more or less
- 2 cups frozen or canned artichoke hearts plain, unmarinated
- 2 cups lowfat cottage cheese

- 8 oz crumbled feta cheese (goat or sheep milk feta is best) - more or less, see note below
- 5 oz fresh spinach roughly chopped
- 3 large eggs divded
- 2 scallions chopped
- 14 cup fresh dill chopped
- 1 tbsp olive oil
- 1 tsp lemon zest
- 12 tsp crushed red pepper flakes
- Salt to taste (as needed)

Direction

Preheat oven to 350 degrees F and grease a 9x9 square baking dish.

If the artichoke hearts are whole, halve them. Heat the olive oil in a large skillet over mediumhigh heat. Sauté the artichokes hearts until browned, then remove from heat and set aside.

Greek Salad Tacos with Cucumber Dill Dressing

Ingridients

- 2 Cups Grilled Chicken
- 4 Cups Cutshredded Romaine Lettuce
- 1 Cup Diced Tomatoes
- 34th Cup Diced Cucumbers
- 14th Cup Diced Cilantro
- 1 Cup Feta Cheese Crumbled

- 12 Cup Sliced Black Olives
- 12 Cup Ken's Greek Dressing
- 1 Cup Dannon Oikos Dips Cucumber and Dill (sold in the refrigerated section with the party dips)
- 8 Flour Tortilla's

Direction

Toss all of the ingredients together for the salad except leave the feta and the cucumber dill dipdressing until you get the salad into the tacos. The cucumber dill dip is made by Dannon and is an Oikos dip that has become a favorite of mine. If you've never tried it before, it's sold in the refrigerated section with the other party dips but its a Greek yogurt dip. If for some reason you cannot find it, you can mix together dill weed, plain greek yogurt and little hint of salt for a similar dip.

If you've never tried a refrigerated tortilla before that has to be cooked, let me tell you that it's life changing. All you have to do is heat them up for about a minute on each side and they are unbelievable good and light. It's all I will use now.

After you toss the salad, fill your tortillas with the salad to make each taco and top with the feta and drizzle of the dip and you are good to go. If you want to make these for dinner and grill your own chicken, the Ken's Greek Dressing is the best marinade for chicken!

Slow Cooker Mediterranean Chicken

Ingredients
- 4 medium-large boneless skinless chicken breasts OR 4-6 boneless skinless chicken thighs
- salt and pepper to taste
- 3 teaspoons Italian seasoning
- juice of 1 medium lemon (about 2 tablespoons)
- 1 tablespoon minced garlic
- 1 medium onion, chopped
- 1 cup kalamata olives
- 1 cup roughly chopped roasted red peppers
- 2 tablespoons capers
- fresh thyme or basil for garnish (optional)

direction

Season chicken with salt and pepper to taste. Cook in a large skillet over medium-high heat 1-2 minutes on each side til browned. Transfer to greased slow cooker.

Add onions, olives, red peppers, and capers to slow cooker (tuck them around the sides so they aren't covering up the chicken). Whisk together italian seasoning, lemon juice, and garlic and pour over chicken.

Cover and cook on low for 4 hours or on high for 2 hours. Garnish with fresh thyme or oregano and serve.

Greek Quesadillas

INGREDIENTS:

- 8 (8-inch) flour tortillas
- 1 (10-ounce) packages frozen chopped spinach, thawed and drained
- 12 cup julienned sun dried tomatoes in olive oil, drained
- 12 cup chopped pitted kalamata olives
- 1 cup shredded mozzarella cheese
- 1 cup crumbled feta cheese
- 1 tablespoon fresh dill

FOR THE TZATZIKI SAUCE

- 1 cup plain Greek yogurt
- 1 English cucumber, finely diced
- 2 cloves garlic, pressed
- 1 tablespoon chopped fresh dill
- 1 tablespoon freshly squeezed lemon juice
- 1 teaspoon lemon zest
- 1 teaspoon chopped fresh mint, optional
- Kosher salt and freshly ground black pepper, to taste
- 2 tablespoons olive oil

DIRECTIONS:

To make the tzatziki sauce, combine Greek yogurt, cucumber, garlic, dill, lemon juice, lemon zest and mint in a small bowl; season with salt and pepper, to taste. Drizzle with olive oil. Refrigerate for at least 10 minutes, allowing the flavors to meld; set aside.

Preheat oven to 400 degrees F. Line a baking sheet with parchment paper.

Top tortilla with spinach, sun dried tomatoes, olives and cheeses, and then top with another tortilla. Repeat with remaining tortillas to make 4 quesadillas.

Place quesadillas onto the prepared baking sheet. Place into oven and bake until the cheese has melted, about 8-10 minutes.

Serve immediately with tzatziki sauce, garnished with dill, if desired.

FLATBREAD PIZZAS WITH WHITE BEAN SPINACH PESTO

Ingredients
- 3 pieces of pita bread or naan (around 78g each)
- 23 cup cannellini beans, or other white beans, drained and rinsed
- 2 cups packed baby spinach
- 1 tablespoon extra-virgin olive oil
- 14 cup natural almonds
- 14 cup fresh basil leaves, torn
- 2 tablespoons water
- 14 teaspoon fine sea salt, plus more for sprinkling
- 18 teaspoon pepper
- 12 cup cherry tomatoes
- 12 cup marinated artichoke hearts
- 12 medium avocado
- 14 small red onion

- 2 ounces crumbled feta cheese with Mediterranean herbs

Directions

Preheat oven to 350°F. Place the pita bread on a baking sheet.

To make the white bean spinach pesto: Combine the white beans, baby spinach, almonds, olive oil, basil, water, sea salt, and pepper in a food processor. Pulse until mostly smooth. Use a spoon to evenly add the pesto to each flatbread.

Halve the cherry tomatoes, chop the artichoke hearts, and thinly slice the avocado and red onion. Evenly arrange on the pizzas.

Sprinkle the feta crumbles evenly onto each flatbread. Finish off the pizzas with a touch of fine sea salt.

Bake the flatbreads for 10 minutes, or until the pita bread is lightly crispy. Allow to cool slightly before using a pizza cutter to slice the flatbreads into 4 slices each.

CHOPPED SALAD

Ingredients
- Meyer Lemon Vinaigrette
- 14 cup Meyer lemon juice
- 14 cup + 2 tablespoons extra-virgin olive oil

- Himalayan pink salt to taste

Chopped Salad

- 12 cup Persian cucumber, chopped
- 12 cup artichoke hearts, chopped
- 12 cup hearts of palm, chopped
- 12 cup tomatoes, chopped
- 2 tablespoons Kalamata olives, chopped
- 2 tablespoons red onion, chopped
- 1 tablespoon capers, chopped
- 12 of an avocado, chopped
- 1 teaspoon fresh basil, chopped

Direction

To make the vinaigrette: Add ingredients to Vitamix or other high-speed blender and blend until emulsified. Adjust salt to taste.

In a large salad bowl, combine cucumber, artichoke hearts, hearts of palm, tomatoes, olives, onion, capers, avocado, and basil.

TOSS SALAD WITH ENOUGH VINAIGRETTE TO COAT EVERYTHING. SERVE AND ENJOY.

Ingredients:

- 4 large eggs
- 4 teaspoons kosher salt

- 8 small Yukon Gold or fingerling potatoes, (about ½ pound)
- 12 pound green beans, trimmed and cut into 1-inch lengths
- For the roasted garlic-lemon vinaigrette:
- 1 tablespoon rice vinegar
- 1 tablespoon fresh lemon juice, preferably Meyer lemon
- 6 tablespoons extra virgin olive oil, grapeseed oil, or sunflower oil, plus more if needed
- 2 to 3 whole basil leaves, cut into thin ribbons
- 2 roasted garlic cloves, minced
- Fresh Kosher salt & freshly ground black pepper

For the salad:

- 1 large head Bibb, butter, or iceberg lettuce, separated into individual leaves
- 1 cup red butter leaves
- 1 cup torn frisee (without tough stems)
- 12 pint cherry tomatoes, halved
- 13 cup pitted Niçoise olives

For the tuna:

- 1 12 tablespoons extra-virgin olive oil
- 2 ahi (yellowfin) tuna fillets or salmon fillets (about 8 ounces each)
- Kosher salt and freshly ground black pepper

Directions:

To cook the eggs and potatoes and blanch the beans:

Place the eggs in a medium saucepan with 2 teaspoons of the salt, cover with water, and bring to a boil. Reduce the heat to medium-low and simmer for 3 minutes. Add the potatoes and simmer with the eggs for 10-12 minutes, until the potatoes are tender. Drain both the eggs and potatoes in a colander and cool in a bowlful of ice and cold water. When the potatoes are cool, remove them from the water bath. Cut Yukon Golds into thick wedges or slice fingerlings lengthwise into quarters. Peel the eggs.

Meanwhile, bring another medium saucepan of water and the remaining 2 teaspoons salt to a boil. Add the beans and boil for 4 minutes, or until crisp-tender. Drain in a colander and cool them in the ice and water, adding more ice if needed. Transfer the beans to a paper-towel-lined plate to cool.

For the vinaigrette:

Pour the vinegar and the lemon juice into a small bowl. Whisking constantly, gradually add the oil in a slow, thin stream until the dressing comes together, adding more oil if necessary. Add the basil, garlic, salt, and pepper to taste. Pour the vinaigrette into a serving cruet and set aside.

For the salad:

Arrange the lettuce leaves on one side of a large platter. Mound the frisee in the center and arrange the tomatoes, olives, potatoes, and green beans in mounds on the platter, leaving space in the center for the tuna on top of the frisee. Cut the eggs into quarters and arrange on the platter.

For the tuna:

Pour the olive oil into a medium skillet or sauté pan and turn the heat to medium-high. When the oil is shimmering but not smoking, add the tuna and sear on one side, 2 to 3 minutes. Turn and sear the other side until cooked through, another 5 to 7 minutes. Transfer to a platter. Stir the vinaigrette and pour a little of it (no more than 3 tablespoons) over the tuna and the salad. Place the remaining vinaigrette on the table so guests can help themselves to more.

To serve, cut the tuna into a few large chunks and then spoon about "2 fingers' worth of into a lettuce leaf cup, along with a little of the eggs, potatoes, frisee, tomatoes, beans, olives, and salt and pepper to taste. Your guests can choose to fold the lettuce around the salad and eat with their hands, or to dig in with a knife and fork.

MEDITERRANEAN NACHOS

Ingredients
- For root vegetable chips:

- 4 beets (mix of colors) andor turnips
- 2 sweet potatoes
- Extra-virgin olive oil
- Kosher salt

For spiced chickpeas:

- 4 tablespoons extra-virgin olive oil, divided
- 1 onion, chopped
- 2 garlic cloves, minced
- 1 12 teaspoons ground cumin
- 1 12 teaspoons smoked paprika
- 1 can chickpeas, drained and rinsed
- 1 cup water
- 12 teaspoon kosher salt

For tahini-yogurt sauce:

- 1 cup unsweetened whole milk yogurt
- 2 tablespoons tahini
- 2 teaspoons fresh lemon juice (14 of a lemon
- 1 garlic clove, grated
- 14 teaspoon kosher salt

Additional ingredients:

- 1 large avocado, diced
- 13 cup feta cheese, crumbled
- 14 cup chopped kalamata or Moroccan olives, pitted
- 2 scallions, green parts thinly sliced
- 2 tablespoons chopped fresh herbs (mint, dill, cilantro, andor parsley)
- Aleppo pepper and flaky sea salt, for finishing

Directions

Preheat oven to 375°F. Scrub root vegetables well and thinly slice with a mandoline. Place sliced vegetables in a bowl; coat with olive oil and season well with salt. (Work with red and yellow beets separately so their color doesn't bleed.)

Arrange sliced vegetables on a sheet pan with a rack placed over top; bake 25 to 30 minutes or until crisp and golden. Alternatively, you can place sliced vegetables directly on sheet pan and turn halfway through.

Meanwhile, make spiced chickpeas: Heat half the olive oil in a saucepan over medium heat. Sauté onions until soft, around 7 to 9 minutes. Add garlic and spices and sauté until fragrant, another minute or so. Add chickpeas, water, and salt. Allow to stew until the chickpeas are soft and most of the water has evaporated, around 20 minutes, stirring occasionally and breaking up chickpeas with a spoon. Stir in remaining olive oil.

To make the yogurt-tahini sauce, whisk all ingredients in a bowl or combine in a blender. (You'll want the sauce to be slightly runny so that you can easily drizzle, so add a tablespoon or two of water if your yogurt is thick.)

To serve, arrange chips on a platter and top with chickpeas, yogurt sauce, and remaining ingredients.

Greek Super Grains Salad with Homemade Pita Chips

Ingredients
- 1 cup mixed quinoa, millet, and buckwheat
- 2 cups water
- salt, to taste
- 3 vine ripe tomatoes, seeded and chopped
- 1 red onion, diced
- 2 small seedless cucumbers, diced
- 1 red bell pepper, seeded and diced
- 1 green bell pepper, seeded and diced
- 1 yellow bell pepper, seeded and diced
- 1 (14 oz) can black olives, drained and sliced
- ½ lb feta, crumbled
- ½ cup olive oil
- 6 tbsp red wine vinegar
- 1 tsp dried oregano
- For the pita chips
- 12 oz mini pitas, quartered
- olive oil, for brushing
- sea salt, for sprinkling

direction
Rinse the grains thoroughly and then drain and place in a medium pot with the water and a few pinches of salt. Bring to a boil and then lower the heat, simmering,

covered, for 15-20 minutes. Remove from the heat and let sit, covered for 5 minutes. Fluff with a fork.

Meanwhile, chop the vegetables and toss them together in a large bowl with the olives and feta. Add the cooked grains to the bowl.

To make the dressing, whisk together the olive oil, vinegar, oregano, and salt, to taste. Toss with the grain mixture.

For the pita chips, heat oven to 375F. Spread the pitas on a parchment-lined baking sheet. Brush with the olive oil and sprinkle with salt. Bake for 12-15 minutes or until crispy.

AVGOLEMONO GREEK LEMON CHICKEN SOUP

INGREDIENTS
- 6 cups chicken stock
- 1 cup orzo
- 3 large eggs
- 14 cup fresh lemon juice
- 1 cup cooked and shredded chicken breast
- Salt and pepper to taste.

Direction
In a large pot, bring chicken stock to a boil.

Add orzo, and cook until al dente.

While the orzo is cooking, whisk together lemon juice and eggs.

When orzo is al dente, ladle out 1 cup of the chicken broth.

Slowly add about 1 tablespoon of broth at a time to the egg mixture, whisking constantly.

Once the broth has been whisked into the egg mixture, slowly stream the egg mixture back into the pot of broth, whisking constantly.

Add the shredded chicken broth, and simmer until soup has thickened, whisking constantly, about 3-5 minutes.

Season with salt and pepper to taste.

SALMON SOUVLAKI BOWLS

INGREDIENTS
SALMON SOUVLAKI

- 1 pound fresh salmon cut into 4 pieces
- 6 tablespoons lemon juice
- 3 tablespoon olive oil
- 2 tablespoons balsamic vinegar
- 1 tablespoon smoked paprika or regular paprika
- 1 tablespoon fresh dill
- 1 tablespoon fresh oregano
- 2 cloves garlic minced or grated

- 12 teaspoon salt
- 1 teaspoon pepper
- BOWLS
- 1 cup dry pearl couscous or farro
- 2 red peppers quartered
- 1 inch zucchini cut into 14 rounds
- 2 tablespoons olive oil
- 1 cup cherry tomatoes halved
- 2 Persian cucumbers sliced
- 12 cup kalamata olives
- 4-8 ounces feta cheese crumbled
- 1 recipe [Tzatziki
- juice from 1 lemon

direction

In a medium sized bowl combine the lemon juice, olive oil, balsamic vinegar, smoked paprika, dill, oregano, garlic, salt and pepper. Add the salmon and toss well, making sure the salmon is completely coated in the seasonings. Let sit for 10-15 minutes.

Meanwhile, cook the couscous or farro according to package directions.

In a bowl, toss together the red peppers, zucchini, 2 tablespoons olive oil, salt + pepper. Toss well to coat the veggies.

Heat your grill, grill pan or skillet to medium high heat.

Transfer the salmon to the preheated grill and grill for about 3 minutes on each side or until the salmon is cooked to your desired doneness. Remove the salmon from the grill. During the same time, add the bell peppers and zucchini, grill 3-4 minutes per side or until char marks appear. Remove everything from the grill.

To assemble, divide the couscous or farro among bowls and drizzle with lemon juice. Add the grilled veggies, salmon, cherry tomatoes, cucumbers, olives and feta cheese. Dollop with Tzatziki and garnish with fresh herbs.

SMOKY VEGAN MOUSSAKA

INGREDIENTS
- TOMATO SAUCE
- 1 (28-ounces) can plum tomatoes
- 1 tablespoon tomato paste
- 1 tsp maple syrup (optional)
- 2 onions, thinly sliced
- 2 garlic cloves, finely chopped
- 12 ounces smoked tofu (firm)
- 18 tsp cinnamon
- 12 tsp salt
- 18 ground black pepper
- a pinch of cayenne pepper
- EGGPLANT
- 3 medium-size eggplants
- 1 tbsp olive oil
- BECHAMEL
- 2 and 12 cups almond milk
- 2 tbsp potato starch

- 2 tbsp nutritional yeast
- 12 tsp salt
- 18 tsp ground nutmeg

Direction

Drain the tomatoes into a bowl. Keep the juice.

Cut the plum tomatoes into small pieces and add to a skillet with their juice.

Heat over medium heat until the sauce thickens, about 10 minutes.

Stir in tomato paste, maple syrup, salt, pepper and cinnamon and remove from heat.

Wash and cut the eggplants into 1-inch think slices, brush slices with olive oil and sprinkle with salt. Fry slices until tender and golden brown on both sides in a large non-stick skillet over medium-heat. Depending on your skillet you can probably fry about 5-6 slices at a time.

Transfer the eggplant slices to paper towels.

Heat one tablespoon of olive oil in a skillet over medium heat. Add the onions and garlic, and cook until soft, about 7 minutes. Scramble the smoked tofu and add to the skillet, cook for about 5 minutes, stirring every 2 minutes. Add the tomato sauce, mix until everything is combined and remove from heat.

Preheat oven to 400°.

Arrange a layer of half the eggplant slices in a greased baking dish (I used a 10-by-6 inch pan). Cover with the tomatotofu sauce. Top with another layer of the remaining eggplant slices.

Pour the bechamel over the top and spread evenly.

Bake 25-30 minutes until top is golden brown.

Top with chopped parsley.

FOR THE BECHAMEL

Add 12 cup almond milk to a medium sauce pan. Mix in the potato starch, nutritional yeast, salt and nutmeg. Whisk until everything is well combined and add the remaining milk. Heat over medium heat for about 5-10 minutes, whisking constantly until it thickens. Remove from heat.

ROASTED CABBAGE STEAKS WITH BASIL PESTO & FETA

Ingredients
- 1 Small Head Cabbage, sliced into "steaks"
- 4 oz Basil Pesto
- 1 cup Shredded Parmesan Cheese
- 2 oz Feta Cheese, crumbled
- 2 small Tomatoes, sliced
- 5-6 Marinated Artichoke halves
- 1 tbsp Mediterranean Seasoning
- Fresh Basil, to garnish
- OPTIONAL TOPPINGS include olives, mozzarella, mushrooms, roasted red pepper, etc.

Direction

Heat oven to 400 and spray a large sheet pan with nonstick spray.

Arrange the cabbage in a single layer on the sheet pan so the edges are all touching. Slather pesto on the steak halves and be generous as a lot will melt into the cabbage folds.

Top with cheese and tomato and bake until the edges of the cabbage are crisp and all of the cheese is bubbly. About 20 minutes.

Sprinkle with Seasoning and Basil. Serve HOT with an extra scoop of Pesto for dipping!

SPANISH GARLIC SHRIMP

Ingredients
- 13 cup olive oil
- 4 cloves garlic, finely chopped
- ¼ teaspoon chili flakes
- 1 pound large shrimp, peeled and deveined
- 1 teaspoon sweet Spanish paprika
- ¼ teaspoon kosher salt
- 18 teaspoon pepper
- 2 tablespoons dry sherry
- 1 ½ tablespoons fresh lemon juice
- 2 tablespoons chopped parsley

Direction

Pour the oil into a large sauté pan and add the garlic and chili flakes. Turn the heat up to medium high. As the pan heats up, the oil will slowly get infused with the flavor of the garlic and chili (do not let the garlic brown). Once the oil is hot and the garlic is fragrant, add the shrimp to the pan. Season them with the paprika, salt and pepper. Cook the shrimp about 2 minutes, until they just turn pink, stirring often. Add the sherry and lemon juice and cook another 2-3 minutes until the liquid is reduced and shrimp are cooked. Sprinkle the parsley on top. Serve with crusty bread for soaking up all of the delicious sauce.

QUINOA STUFFED EGGPLANT WITH TAHINI SAUCE

Ingredients
- 1 eggplant
- 2 tablespoons olive oil divided
- 1 medium shallot diced (about 12 cup)
- 1 cup chopped button mushrooms about 2 cups whole
- 5 - 6 Tuttorosso whole plum tomatoes chopped
- 1 tablespoon tomato juice from the can
- 2 garlic cloves minced
- 12 cup cooked quinoa
- 12 teaspoon ground cumin
- 1 tablespoon chopped fresh parsley + more to garnish

- Salt & pepper to taste
- 1 tablespoon tahini
- 1 teaspoon lemon juice
- 12 teaspoon garlic powder
- Water to thin

Direction

Preheat the oven to 425ºF. Cut the eggplant in half lengthwise and scoop out some of the flesh. Place on a baking sheet and drizzle with 1 tablespoon of oil. Sprinkle with salt and bake for 20 minutes.

While the eggplant is cooking, heat the remaining oil in a large skillet. Once add all the shallots and mushrooms. Saute until mushrooms have softened, about 5 minutes. Add tomatoes, quinoa and spices, and cook until the liquid has evaporated.

Once the eggplant has cooked for 20 minutes, reduce the oven temperature to 350ºF and stuff each half with the tomato-quinoa mixture. Bake for another 10 minutes.

When ready to serve, whisk together tahini, lemon, garlic, water and a touch of salt and pepper. Drizzle tahini over eggplants, sprinkle with parsley and enjoy!

CROCK POT CHICKEN THIGHS WITH ARTICHOKES AND SUN-DRIED TOMATOES

Ingredients

- 4 to 6 boneless chicken thighs
- salt and fresh ground pepper , to taste
- 12 tablespoon dried oregano
- 1 jar (14.75-ounces) Cara Mia Grilled Artichoke Hearts, drained, 13-cup liquid reserved
- 1 bag (3.5-ounces) Julienne Cut Sun-Dried Tomatoes
- 4 cloves garlic , minced
- 13- cup artichoke hearts liquid
- 3 tablespoons chopped fresh parsley

Direction

Spray 5 to 6-quart crock potslow cooker with cooking spray.

Season chicken thighs with salt, pepper, and dried oregano; add to slow cooker in one layer.

Add artichoke hearts and sun-dried tomatoes over the chicken; sprinkle with garlic.

Take a 13-cup of the liquid from the jar with the artichoke hearts and pour it over the top.

Cover; cook on HIGH for 4 to 4-12 hours, or on LOW for about 6 hours.

Transfer to serving plates.

Sprinkle with fresh parsley.

Serve.

Bowtie Pasta with Sausage and Escarole

Ingredients
- 6 ounces uncooked bowtie pasta
- 14 teaspoon table salt
- 1 teaspoon olive oil
- 8 ounces uncooked turkey sausage, hot italian variety, castings removed 1 small uncooked onions, chopped 4 medium garlic cloves, sliced
- 1 small uncooked onions, chopped
- 4 medium garlic cloves, sliced
- 8 cups escarole, roughly chopped in bite-size pieces
- 34 cup canned chicken broth
- 14 12 ounces canned fire-roasted diced tomatoes
- 1 teaspoon crushed red pepper flakes, or to taste
- 14 cup grated Parmesan cheese

Direction

Cook pasta in lightly salted water according to package directions; drain pasta and return to pot.

Meanwhile, heat oil in a large nonstick skillet over medium-high heat. Add sausage and onion; cook, breaking up sausage as it cooks, until sausage is lightly browned, about 5 minutes.

Add garlic, escarole, and broth to skillet; cook, stirring often, until escarole is tender, about 5 minutes. Stir in tomatoes and red pepper flakes; cook until heated through, about 1 minute.

Spoon sauce over pasta; toss to coat. Sprinkle with cheese; sprinkle with red pepper flakes (if desired).

SPICY GREEK LAYERED DIPS

Ingredients
- 1 cup tzatziki sauce
- 1 teaspoon minced garlic
- 1 cup minced red onion
- 1 cup roasted red peppers (packed in water), chopped
- 12 tablespoons spicy or regular hummus
- 1 cup diced cucumber
- 1 cup chopped plum tomato
- 10 large Kalamata olive, chopped
- 4 tablespoons crumbled feta cheese
- 14 cup fresh mint leaves

Direction
In a small bowl, combine tzatziki with garlic.

Line up eight 9-oz plastic cups (or small glass cups or bowls). In each cup, layer 2 tablespoons tzatziki mixture, 2 tablespoons onion, 2 tablespoons pepper, 1 12 tablespoons hummus, 2 tablespoons cucumber, 2 tablespoons tomato, 1 tablespoon olives and 12 tablespoon feta; garnish with mint. Refrigerate until ready to serve.

Roasted Moroccan Chicken with Spinach Salad

Ingredients
- 12 cup olive oil
- 1 12 teaspoons cumin
- 1 12 teaspoons coriander
- 1 12 teaspoons paprika
- 1 12 teaspoons yellow curry powder
- 12 teaspoon crushed red pepper flakes
- 3 garlic cloves
- 1 tablespoon grated ginger
- 4 teaspoons lemon juice
- 1 bunches parsley (including stems), roughly chopped
- Kosher salt
- Black pepper
- 1 small whole chicken (about 3 pounds)
- 6 cups spinach
- 2 tablespoons capers
- 14 small red onion, thinly sliced
- 1 tablespoon extra virgin olive oil
- 14 cup pecorino

Direction

Preheat the oven to 400 degrees . Prepare marinade: Add olive oil, cumin, coriander, paprika, curry powder, red pepper flakes, garlic, ginger, and 1 teaspoon lemon juice to a blender and blend for 1 minute on low. Add parsley and blend until smooth and bright green. Season to taste with salt and pepper.

Use kitchen twine to truss the chicken if desired, tucking the wings under the bird and tying the legs together. Rub chicken with marinade. Transfer to oven and roast until internal temperature reaches 165 degrees at the thickest part of the thigh, 45 minutes to 1 hour.

When chicken is done, let rest for 5 minutes. Prepare salad: Toss spinach, capers, and red onion with remaining 1 tablespoon lemon juice and extra-virgin olive oil. Top with pecorino. Serve the chicken with the salad.

Whole wheat penne with roasted tomatoes, asparagus, and leeks

Ingredients
- Cooking spray
- 2 pounds uncooked asparagus
- 2 medium uncooked leeks
- 6 cups cherry fresh ingredients
- 2 tablespoons extra virgin olive oil
- 1 teaspoon kosher salt, or to taste
- 14 teaspoon black pepper

- 8 ounces uncooked whole wheat pasta, penne
- table salt
- 12 cup chopped basil
- 1 teaspoon minced garlic
- 1 teaspoon lemon zest
- cup shredded Parmigiano Reggiano cheese

direction

Preheat oven to 375 degrees F. Coat 2 baking sheets with cooking spray.

Cut leeks lengthwise and soak in a bowl of water; rinse well to remove dirt and cut white and light green parts into1-inch pieces. Trim asparagus; cut into 1-inch pieces.

Toss asparagus, leeks, and tomatoes with oil, kosher salt, and pepper; spread evenly on prepared baking sheets. Roast, stirring once halfway through, about 35 to 40 minutes.

Meanwhile, bring a large pot of salted water to a boil. Cook penne according to package instructions; reserve 14 cup pasta cooking water and then drain pasta.

In a serving bowl, toss together penne, cooking water, roasted vegetables, basil, garlic, and lemon zest; garnish with Parmesan.

FARRO HERB SALAD WITH CHICKEN

Ingredients

- 2 chicken breasts, boneless and skinless
- Salt and pepper
- 3 tablespoons extra virgin olive oil, divided
- 1⁄2 cup basil, packed
- 1⁄2 cup mint, packed
- 1⁄2 cup parsley, packed
- 1 nectarine
- 1⁄2 cup cherries, pitted
- 1⁄2 avocado
- 1⁄2 cup chickpeas
- 1 cup quinoa, cooked
- 2 cups farro, cooked
- 1⁄2 teaspoon dijon mustard
- Juice of 1 lemon
- Zest of 1⁄2 lemon

Directions

Preheat oven to 400 degrees F.

Heat 1 tablespoon olive oil in a large ovenproof skillet. Season chicken breasts generously with salt and pepper. When pan is hot, add chicken breasts. After 2 minutes, flip chicken breasts and cook on the other side for 3 minutes. Place pan in the oven and cook for 10 to 15 minutes or until a meat thermometer registers 165 degrees F.

Meanwhile, slice all herbs into thin ribbons and place in a large bowl. Chop nectarine, cherries and avocado into small cubes and add to the herbs along with chickpeas and feta.

In a small bowl, whisk together dijon, lemon juice and lemon zest until smooth. Add remaining 2 tablespoons of oil in a slow stream, whisking quickly and consistently to combine.

Gently fold the quinoa, farro and dressing into the herb mixture. Season with salt and pepper.

Slice the chicken breasts thinly.

Evenly distribute the farro salad between 4 dishes and top with 12 chicken breast.

OPEN-FACED CHICKEN BRUSCHETTA SANDWICHES

Ingredients
- 4 slices whole grain bread or 1 whole wheat baguette, sliced
- 2 teaspoons olive oil
- 4 thin slices mozzarella cheese
- 1 pound skinless, boneless chicken breast cutlets
- Salt and pepper to taste
- 1 tablespoon canola oil
- 2 teaspoons Italian seasoning
- 3 roma tomatoes, chopped
- 13 red onion, chopped
- 1 clove garlic, chopped
- 2 teaspoons olive oil
- 1 teaspoon balsamic vinegar
- 14 cup fresh basil, chopped

Direction

Preheat oven to 425 degrees F. Place the bread on a baking sheet and drizzle with the oil. Place the bread in the oven and cook for 3-5 minutes, or to desired crispness.

For the chicken, add the oil and seasonings and set aside. Heat a grill, Panini press, or skillet over medium high heat. Cook for 3-4 minutes per side or until the chicken is cooked through.

While the chicken and bread are cooking, assemble the bruschetta by combining the tomatoes, onion, garlic, oil, balsamic vinegar, and basil in a bowl. Mix well.

To assemble the sandwiches, top each slice of bread with 1-2 chicken cutlets (depending on size), then place a slice of cheese over the chicken. Just before serving, top each sandwich with the bruschetta.

VEGETABLE LENTIL SOUP

INGREDIENTS
- 2 tablespoons olive oil
- 1 small onion, diced
- 2 large carrots, peeled and chopped
- 5 cloves garlic, minced
- 2 teaspoons cumin
- 12 teaspoon dried thyme
- 2 (15 oz) cans fire roasted diced tomatoes
- 1 (15 oz) can chickpeas, drained and rinsed

- 1 cup green lentils
- 1 (1 quart) box Progresso vegetable cooking stock
- 3 cups water
- 1 teaspoon salt
- 1 teaspoon pepper
- 12 teaspoon red pepper flakes
- 2 cups kale, ribs removed and chopped

Direction

Heat olive oil in a large stock pot over medium heat. Add the onions and carrots, cook stirring often, until onion becomes tender and translucent.

Add the garlic, cumin, and thyme. Cook until fragrant. Add fire roasted tomatoes and chickpeas.

Add the lentils, then pour in Progresso vegetable cooking stock and water. Season with salt, pepper and red pepper flakes. Bring soup to a boil, then turn down to a gentle simmer. Cook for 30 minutes, until the lentils are tender.

Transfer 3 cups of soup into a blender or food processor (make sure to get an even mixture of veggies and broth). Puree mixture until smooth. Add pureed soup back into the pot and add kale. Cook until wilted.

SPINACH FETA GRILLED CHEESE

INGREDIENTS
- 12 Tbsp olive oil

- 1 clove garlic
- 14 lb frozen cut spinach
- Pinch of salt and pepper
- 2 ciabatta rolls
- 1 cup shredded mozzarella cheese
- 1 oz feta cheese
- pinch red pepper flakes (optional)

direction

Mince the garlic and add it to a skillet with the olive oil. Cook over medium-low heat for 1-2 minutes, or until it begins to soften. Add the frozen spinach, turn the heat up to medium, and cook for about 5 minutes, or until heated through and most of the excess moisture has evaporated away. Season lightly with salt and pepper.

Cut the rolls in half. Add about 14 cup of shredded mozzarella and 12 oz. of feta to the bottom half of each roll. Divide the cooked spinach between the two sandwiches, then top with a pinch of red pepper flakes, plus 14 more shredded mozzarella on each.

Place the top half of the ciabatta roll on the sandwiches and transfer them to a large non-stick skillet. Fill a large pot with a few inches of water to create weight, then place the pot on top of the sandwiches to press them down like a panini press. Turn the heat on to medium-low and cook until the sandwiches are crispy on the bottom. Carefully flip the sandwiches, place the weighted pot back on top, and cook until crispy on the other side and the cheese is melted. Serve warm

Quinoa Tabbouleh

ingredients
- 1 cup quinoa (170 g)
- 2 cups water (500 g)
- ½ cup chopped spring onion (50 g)
- 1⅓ cup chopped tomatoes (240 g)
- 1 cup finely chopped fresh mint (26 g) ½ cup finely chopped fresh parsley (30 g)
- The juice of a lemon
- Extra virgin olive oil to taste (optional)

Direction

Rinse the quinoa with cool water.

Boil the water in a saucepan, add the quinoa and simmer for about 15 minutes or until all the water has been absorbed. You can add other ingredients (dried herbs, sea salt, tamari or soy sauce, lemon juice or apple cider vinegar) to the boiling water to get a more intense flavor.

Let the quinoa cool at room temperature, or add cold water. It has to be completely cool before making the salad.

In a large bowl, place the quinoa and the rest of the ingredients. Add the lemon juice and the extra virgin olive oil (optional) and stir.

Garlic and Anchovy Roasted Lamb Chops with a Castelvetrano & Sage Browned Butter Sauce

Ingredients:

- 3 garlic cloves, minced
- 2 anchovy fillets, minced
- 1 teaspoon anchovy oil
- 12 teaspoon cracked black pepper
- 6 American Lamb Chops, room temperature
- 2 tablespoons extra virgin olive oil
- 14 cup (12stick) unsalted butter
- 10 castelvetrano olives, pitted and chopped
- 8 fresh sage leaves
- salt and pepper to taste

Directions:

Preheat oven to 375°F.

Place garlic, anchovies, anchovy oil, and black pepper in a small bowl and whisk together.

Lightly season lamb chops with salt and pepper.

Brush garlic-anchovy mixture over each chop, on both sides.

Pour olive oil into a large sauté pan and place over medium-high heat.

Sear each chop in the pan for 2 to 3 minutes, on each side, and transfer to a roasting pan.

Roast lamb chops for about 13 to 15 minutes for medium-rare, and 15 to 18 minutes for medium doneness. Remove from the oven and allow chops to rest for 5 to 7 minutes.

Using the same pan you used to sear the chops, melt the butter over medium-low heat. Allow butter to cook for 6 to 8 minutes or until butter has melted and begins to foam and brown. Add olives and sage leaves and gently fry for 1 to 2 minutes. Remove mixture from the heat. Season with salt and pepper.

Transfer chops onto a serving dishplatter and pour butter sauce over chops. Serve immediately.

CANDIED GRAPE AND CHERRY TOMATOES WITH BAKED FETA

Ingredients
- 2 tablespoons extra-virgin olive oil, divided
- 2 pints multicolored grape and cherry tomatoes
- 1 tablespoon balsamic vinegar
- 1 garlic clove, minced
- 14 teaspoon kosher salt
- 1 (4-ounce) block feta, cut into thin slabs
- 12 cup sunflower or other sprouts
- 1 tablespoon sliced fresh basil leaves
- Coarsely ground black pepper

Direction

Preheat oven to 400 degrees F. Brush an 8 x 8-inch glass or ceramic baking dish with 1 tablespoon oil. Arrange feta in a single layer.

In a large high-sided skillet, heat remaining 1 tablespoon oil over medium heat. Add tomatoes and cook, stirring often, until tomatoes begin to burst, 10 to 15 minutes. Stir in balsamic vinegar, garlic, and salt. Cook until liquid has thickened, about 5 minutes.

While tomatoes are cooking, bake feta until springy to the touch but not melted, 12 to 15 minutes.

To serve, divide feta among serving plates and spoon tomatoes with cooking liquid on top. Garnish with sprouts, basil, and black pepper.

WALNUT-ROSEMARY CRUSTED SALMON

Ingredients
- 2 teaspoons Dijon mustard
- 1 clove garlic, minced
- ¼ teaspoon lemon zest
- 1 teaspoon lemon juice
- 1 teaspoon chopped fresh rosemary
- ½ teaspoon honey
- ½ teaspoon kosher salt
- ¼ teaspoon crushed red pepper
- 3 tablespoons panko breadcrumbs
- 3 tablespoons finely chopped walnuts
- 1 teaspoon extra-virgin olive oil
- 1 (1 pound) skinless salmon fillet, fresh or frozen

- Olive oil cooking spray

Direction

Preheat oven to 425°F. Line a large rimmed baking sheet with parchment paper. Combine mustard, garlic, lemon zest, lemon juice, rosemary, honey, salt and crushed red pepper in a small bowl. Combine panko, walnuts and oil in another small bowl. Place salmon on the prepared baking sheet. Spread the mustard mixture over the fish and sprinkle with the panko mixture, pressing to adhere. Lightly coat with cooking spray. Bake until the fish flakes easily with a fork, about 8 to 12 minutes, depending on thickness.

MEDITERRANEAN MEAL SHOPPING LIST IDEAS

You have the knowledge, you have the recipes now it's time to put everything to the test. First, set yourself up for success by stocking your pantry with best Mediterranean diet foods, from the healthiest seafood to the healthiest nuts and seeds. Next time you visit the grocery store or farmers' market, refer to this handy shopping list.

- Vegetable Ideas

- Kale, Swiss chard, arugula
- Leeks, onions, shallots, garlic
- Radishes, beets, carrots
- Sweet potatoes
- Cucumbers
- Artichokes
- Fennel
- Eggplant
- Peppers
- Protein Ideas
- Canned tuna, salmon, or anchovies
- Fresh salmon or mackerel, oysters, mussels
- Eggs
- Lean game meats such as quail, duck, and bison
- Fat Ideas
- Extra-virgin olive oil
- Canola oil
- Safflower oil
- Whole Grain Ideas
- Quinoa
- Farro
- Bulgur
- Barley
- Wheat Berries
- Nut and Seed Ideas
- Almonds, pine nuts, walnuts
- Sesame seeds
- Dairy Ideas
- Feta, goat cheese, haloumi, ricotta, Parmigiano-Reggiano

- Greek yogurt
- Fruit Ideas
- Olives, avocados, tomatoes,
- Figs, apricots, dates
- Pears, oranges, grapes, cherries, pomegranates
- Legumes
- Chickpeas, cannellini beans, fava beans
- Lentils, split peas
- Peanuts
- Condiments and Spices
- Tahini
- Harissa
- Fig spread
- Hummus, tapenade, pesto,
- Za'atar
- Ground cumin, turmeric, ground coriander, Spanish paprika (also called pimentón)
- Saffron threads

Conclusion

During the past twenty years, a significant number of people in different countries around the world have turned their attention towards finding healthy diet regimens that are low in saturated fat and that include bountiful servings of fresh fruits and vegetable. Consequently, the Mediterranean diet has caught the eye of innumerable people who want to include healthy eating into their overall course of prudent living. In short, the Mediterranean diet encompasses foods and beverages that, when consumed in moderation, can work to lessen the threat of some serious diseases and can aid in creating the necessary foundation for a long, hearty lifetime.

Prime constituents Mediterranean diet predominantly consists of fibers such as grains, fruit, beans and vegetables. Fibers in pasta, rice, bread, bulgur (dried cracked wheat), polenta, potatoes and couscous, are natural fillers and so prevent a person from periodically reaching out for snacks. Researchers also feel that the liberal consumption of yogurt and garlic have beneficial effects.

The Mediterranean diet also involves limited consumption of red meat. This avoidance of high calorie foods clearly helps, not just with maintaining healthy weight but with weight loss as well. Some researchers argue that the large amount of fish, fruit and nuts consumed in the diet provide anti-oxidants that delay the appearance of wrinkles and helps as an anti-aging method.

Not a new-fangled technique: It is interesting to note that the 'Mediterranean Diet' is less a new-fangled technique to maintain healthy weight and more a result of health-conscious people re-looking at eating habits that have been followed in the Mediterranean region for thousands of years. Thus the Mediterranean Diet promotes a radically different perspective on 'food' and 'consumption' and is less of a 'diet' to be tried for a short duration of time, and more a way of life that one can choose to adopt permanently.

A Mediterranean Diet meal plan is very easy to follow because the food selection includes full flavor fats, whole breads and cereals, fruits, vegetables, nuts, seeds, beans, and a host of out hunger blasting foods. But perhaps the best benefit of following a Mediterranean Diet meal plan is how effective it is at dropping pounds of dangerous belly fat.

Where you carry your extra pounds of fat can make a big difference in your overall health picture. Too much belly fat causes your internal organs to be crowded and this causes a chain reaction of poor health consequences from increased LDL (bad) cholesterol levels to high blood pressure, diabetes, and heart disease.

If you take a tape measure and wrap it around your belly at the level just above your hip bones and it measures more than 40 inches if you are a man or more than 35 inches if you are a woman, that means you need a healthy shift in your diet and following a Mediterranean Diet meal plan may be the answer.

I like to think of the Mediterranean Diet meal plan as the Food Pyramid turned up side down and shuffled. What I mean is that the Mediterranean Diet meal plan puts less emphasis on meats and more emphasis on monounsaturated and polyunsaturated fats, fruits, vegetables and whole grains.

The Mediterranean Diet meal plan is more a way of eating rather than a diet. In fact, when researchers refer to the Mediterranean Diet, they are referring to the lifestyle of people in a regions of the world that border the Mediterranean Sea such as Greece, Italy, France, Spain, and Morocco.

You can follow a Mediterranean Diet meal plan or you can create your own meals based on the core food items. For instance, you may start your day with fruits or at times an egg omelet with vegetables, snack throughout the day on nuts, seeds, and legumes, and feast at lunch and dinner on robust salads, fish or white meat.

The combinations of foods on a Mediterranean Diet meal plan are endless making this a great diet for the creative cook.

Following a Mediterranean Diet meal plan is a safe way to lose belly fat as well as fat from other areas of your body. The diet is naturally high in fiber, vitamins, antioxidants, and minerals, which means your heart is protected as you lose weight. Isn't that a better side effect than taking a weight loss drug?

Is your belly too big? Are you worried that you have let your weight go too far and now feel stressed and anxious about what in the world you are going to do to get rid of this belly fat?

I know how scary this can be and what I don't want you to do is jump on the band wagon of some silly fat diet that promises super fast fat loss, but ends up leaving you feeling tired, moody, and absolutely starving.

Part 2

INTRODUCTION

One of the trendy diets that have gained some attention is the Eat-Clean Diet. The Eat-Clean Diet is "a lifestyle way of eating that allows you to eat more, weigh less, and become the healthiest you can be." We will look for the positives and negatives of this diet, and how it would fit with a proper diet for the average person trying to lose weight on a long-term basis.

This diet is rich in plant food, including whole grains, fruits, vegetables, and lean proteins, nonfat dairy, and healthy organic fats. Their emphasis on good health and weight loss is 80% food, 10% exercise, and 10% genes. Cornerstones of the plan are regular exercise and a calorie-controlled diet high in fiber, with lean protein to satisfy hunger on fewer calories.

A nutritious breakfast with high fiber carbohydrates, lean protein and some healthy fat throughout the day will boost metabolism. Each meal during the day should be between 200-300 calories, a complex carbohydrate with protein should be part of every meal, and drink at least eight cups of water daily. Add weight training and physical activity a minimum of three days a week for about 30 minutes, and you should lose about three pounds a week. So far, we would agree with everything they say.

Exercising, consuming fruits, vegetables and lean meats while controlling portion sizes, and exercising is the recommendation of any credible diet. Also, the total elimination of artificial ingredients, preservatives, sugars, and Tran's fat no credible dietician would disagree with. But we disagree with the total elimination of saturated fat, foods "whose ingredients you can't pronounce", the elimination of alcohol except perhaps a once a week glass of red wine. We also disagree with the part about bringing your food when to avoid eating in restaurants.

There must be more latitude to cheat on your diet, or only those willing to live the most Spartan lifestyle will be able to maintain it over the long-term. Dining out occasionally is a social experience, and for any program to ask you to eliminate that would be asking quite a lot. Instead, work the dining out experience with eating healthy, portion-controlled food, and if the portions are too large have the discipline to take the surplus home. The healthy-cooking methods described here best capture the flavor and retain the nutrients in foods without adding excessive amounts of fat or salt. Use them often to prepare your favorite dishes.

<u>Baking</u>

Besides bread and desserts, you can bake seafood, poultry, lean meat, vegetables and fruits. For baking, place food in a pan or dish, covered or uncovered. Baking generally doesn't require that you add fat to the food.

<u>Sauteing</u>

Sauteing quickly cooks relatively small or thin pieces of food. If you choose a good-quality nonstick pan, you can cook food without using fat. Depending on the recipe, use low-sodium broth, cooking spray or water in place of oil.

Stir-frying

A traditional Asian method, stir-frying quickly cooks small, uniform-sized pieces of food while they're rapidly stirred in a wok or large nonstick frying pan. You need only a small amount of oil or cooking spray for this cooking method.

Steaming

One of the simplest cooking techniques is steaming food in a perforated basket suspended above simmering liquid. If you use a flavorful liquid or add seasonings to the water, you'll flavor the food as it cooks.

Roasting

Like baking, but typically at higher temperatures, roasting uses an oven's dry heat to cook the food. You can roast foods on a baking sheet or in a roasting pan.

For poultry, seafood and meat, place a rack inside the roasting pan so that the fat in the food can drip away during cooking. To maintain moisture, cook foods until they reach a safe internal temperature but don't overcook them.

New Ways To Flavor Foods

Creating meals with herbs, spices and other natural flavorings is one of the best ways to add color, taste and aroma to foods without adding salt or fat. Healthy flavor boosts include:

Fresh herbs. Choose herbs that look bright and aren't wilted, and add them toward the end of cooking.

Dried herbs. Add pinches of dried herbs in the earlier stages of cooking. But avoid prepackaged seasoning mixes because they often contain more of salt.

Dried mustard. Used sparingly, dried mustard adds a zesty flavor while cooking.

Vinegar or citrus juices. Add them at the last moment. Vinegar is great on vegetables, and citrus works well on fruit such as melons.

Marinades. Try an low-fat marinade for foods that you broil, grill or roast. To make your own marinade, use 1 part oil to 2 parts vinegar or citrus juice, and add herbs and spices as desired.

Fresh hot peppers. Remove the membranes and seeds first, and then finely chop the peppers. A small amount goes a long way.

Dried vegetables and fruits. Some vegetables and fruits — such as mushrooms, tomatoes, chilies, cherries, cranberries, and currants — have a more intense flavor when dried than when fresh. Add them when you want a burst of flavor.

CHAPTER ONE

THE LIST OF TRENDING RECIPE

RAITHA WITH CUCUMBER (KHEERA)

Prep time: 5 minutes
Serving Per: 5 serves
Cooking time: None
Calories: 37

Ingredients
- [ ] 10cm4in cucumber
- [ ] 300g10 12 oz low-fat natural yogurt
- [ ] 12 teaspoon cumin, roasted, and ground
- [ ] 12 teaspoon black pepper, coarsely ground
- [ ] 12 teaspoon coriander, finely chopped

Directions
Sweet potato curry with spinach and chick peas
Split mung dhal (dry dhal)
Peel and grate the cucumber and mix it with the yoghurt.
Add the cumin, black pepper and coriander.
Mix well and serve as a side dish.Pork Tenderloin with Seasoned Rub

Nutritional Info

- Total Fat: 0.7g   1 %
- Saturated Fat: 0.4g   2 %
- Energy (kcal): 37   2 %
- Sugar: 4.1g   5 %
- Salt: 0.11g   2 %

GARLIC BUTTER STEAK BITES WITH ZUCCHINI NOODLES MEAL PREP

Seared steak bites are tossed in a flavorful garlic butter sauce and served with garlic butter flavored zucchini noodles. This is an easy dish that comes together in minutes and can be made ahead of time for weekly meal prep.

Prep Time: 15 Minutes
Cook Time: 15 Minutes
Total Time: 30 Minutes
Serving Per:4 serves

Ingredients

- [ ] 3 teaspoons butter
- [ ] 6 cloves garlic minced
- [ ] 1 teaspoon low sodium soy sauce
- [ ] 12 teaspoon garlic powder
- [ ] 1 teaspoon canola oil or olive oil

- ☐ 1 lb of sirloin steak cut into bite size pieces
- ☐ salt to taste
- ☐ 1 teaspoon parsley chopped
- ☐ 4 large zucchini spiralized

Directions

In a small saucepan, add butter and garlic. Cook over low medium heat until butter is melted and garlic starts to brown and the flavor of the garlic is infused with the butter. Stir in the garlic powder and soy sauce. Taste and adjust as needed. Set aside.

Add the canola oil to a large cast iron skillet and bring to high heat. When oil is hot, add in the steak.

Cook steak about 1-2 minutes on each side, letting them develop a golden sear before flipping them. Lightly season steak with salt as needed. (Keep in mind that the sauce will add sodium to the steak).

When steak is almost finished cooking, pour two-thirds of the garlic butter sauce over the steak. Stir steak until it is cooked and evenly coated in the sauce. Garnish with parsley.

Remove steak from pan and divide into meal prep containers.

Using the same pan (and keeping in any remaining sauces from the steak and sauce), add in the zucchini noodles and remaining garlic butter sauce. Stir zucchini noodles until they are fully cooked. Season with salt as needed. Drain water from zucchini noodles and then add to meal prep containers.

Nutrition Info

- Total Fat 18g 28%
- Saturated Fat 7g 35%
- Cholesterol 92mg 31%
- Sodium 291mg 12%
- Potassium 917mg 26%
- Total Carbohydrates 8g 3%
- Dietary Fiber 2g 8%
- Sugars 5g
- Protein 27g 54%
- Vitamin A 14.8%
- Vitamin C 45.8%
- Calcium 7.4%
- Iron 15.5%

CREAMY STRAWBERRY-PINEAPPLE SMOOTHIE

Prep Time: 10 minutes
Serving Per:2 servings
Ready In:10 minutes
Calories: 138

Ingredients
- ☐ 12 cup pineapple juice
- ☐ 12 cup plain low-fat yogurt

- [ ] 12 cup halved strawberries1 banana (optional)

Directions

Blend pineapple juice, yogurt, strawberries, and banana together in a blender until smooth.

Nutrition Info

- Total Fat: 1.3g   2 %
- Saturated Fat: 1.0g
- Cholesterol: 4mg   1 %
- Sodium: 45mg   2 %
- Potassium: 499mg   14 %
- Total Carbohydrates: 29g   9 %
- Dietary Fiber: 2.5g   10 %
- Protein: 4.4g   9 %

MANGO LIME SMOOTHIE

Prep Time: 10 minutes
Serving Per: 4 servings
Ready In: 10 minutes
Calories: 117

Ingredients

- [ ] 3 mangoes, peeled, pitted, and cut into 1-inch chunks
- [ ] 2 tablespoons fresh lime juice
- [ ] 2 tablespoons confectioners' sugar
- [ ] 1 tray ice cubes

Directions

Place the mangoes, lime juice, confectioners' sugar, and ice cubes in a blender. Blend until slushy.

Nutrition Info

- Total Fat: 0.4g < 1 %
- Saturated Fat: 0.0g
- Cholesterol: 0mg   0 %
- Sodium: 6mg   < 1 %
- Potassium: 252mg   7 %
- Total Carbohydrates: 30.7g   10 %
- Dietary Fiber: 2.8g   11 %
- Protein: 0.8g   2 %
- Sugars: 27g
- Vitamin A: 1192IU
- Vitamin C: 45mg

COCONUT OIL COFFEE

Prep Time:5 minutes
Serving Per:2 servings
Ready In :5 minutes
Calories: 224

Ingredients

☐   2 cups hot coffee
☐   2 tablespoons coconut oil
☐   2 tablespoons unsalted butter

Directions

Blend coffee, coconut oil, and butter together in a blender until oil and butter are melted and coffee is frothy.

Nutrition Info

- Total Fat: 25.6g 39 %
- Saturated Fat: 20.0g
- Cholesterol: 31mg 10 %
- Sodium: 6mg < 1 %
- Potassium: 120mg 3 %
- Total Carbohydrates: 0g   < 1 %
- Dietary Fiber: 0g 0 %
- Protein: 0.4g   < 1 %
- Sugars: 0g
- Vitamin A: 355IU
- Vitamin C: 0mg
- Folate: 5mcg

CHAPTER TWO

QUICK START BREAKFAST DRINK

Prep Time: 10 minutes
Serving Per: 4 servings
Ready In: 10 minutes
Calories: 263

Ingredients

- ☐ 2 cups pineapple juice
- ☐ 2 bananas
- ☐ 2 cups vanilla yogurt1 cup strawberries, hulled
- ☐ 14 cup wheat germ
- ☐ 1 teaspoon vanilla extract
- ☐ Add all ingredients to list

Directions

In a blender combine pineapple juice, bananas yogurt, strawberries, wheat germ and vanilla extract. Blend until smooth.

Nutrition Info

- Total Fat: 2.7g   4 %
- Saturated Fat: 1.0g
- Cholesterol: 6mg   2 %
- Sodium: 85mg   3 %
- Potassium: 763mg   21 %
- Total Carbohydrates: 53.1g   17 %
- Dietary Fiber: 3.5g   14 %

- Protein: 9g   18 %
- Sugars: 38g
- Vitamin A: 101IU
- Vitamin C: 40mg
- Calcium: 237mg
- Iron: 1mg
- Thiamin: 0mg
- Niacin: 3mg
- Vitamin B6: 1mg
- Magnesium: 73mg
- Folate: 77mcg

CARROT AND ORANGE JUICE

Prep Time: 10 minutes
Serving Per: 4 servings
Ready In:10 minutes
Calories: 183

Ingredients
☐   2 pounds organic carrots, trimmed and scrubbed
☐   8 organic oranges, peeled

Directions

Press carrots and oranges through a juicer and into a large glass.

Nutrition Info
- Total Fat: 0.8g   1 %

- Saturated Fat: 0.0g
- Cholesterol: 0mg 0 %
- Sodium: 157mg   6 %
- Potassium: 1074mg   30 %
- Total Carbohydrates: 44.3g   14 %
- Dietary Fiber: 11g   44 %
- Protein: 3.9g   8 %
- Sugars: 29g
- Vitamin A: 38355IU
- Vitamin C: 116mg
- Calcium: 152mg
- Iron: 1mg
- Thiamin: 0mg
- Niacin: 3mg
- Vitamin B6: 0mg
- Magnesium: 46mg
- Folate: 101mcg

GINGERBREAD LATTE SYRUP

"This gingerbread latte syrup is super quick to make and has great authentic gingerbread flavor. To serve, add 2 to 3 tablespoons of the gingerbread syrup to 8 ounces of hot milk mixed with 2 ounces of hot espresso. Store in the fridge in an airtight container."
Prep Time: 5 minutes
Serving Per: 12 servings

Ready In: 5 minutes
Calories: 63

Ingredients

- ☐ 23 cup agave nectar
- ☐ 1 tablespoon molasses
- ☐ 1 tablespoon ground ginger
- ☐ 2 teaspoons vanilla extract
- ☐ 12 teaspoon ground cinnamon
- ☐ 2 pinches ground cloves
- ☐ 2 pinches salt

Directions

Whisk agave, molasses, ginger, vanilla extract, cinnamon, cloves, and salt in a bowl until well-mixed, about 2 minutes.

Nutrition Info

- Total Fat: 0.1g < 1 %
- Saturated Fat: 0.0g
- Cholesterol: 0mg 0 %
- Sodium: 27mg 1 %
- Potassium: 34mg < 1 %
- Total Carbohydrates: 16.1g 5 %
- Dietary Fiber: 1.1g 4 %
- Protein: 0.1g < 1 %
- Sugars: 14g
- Vitamin A: 2IU
- Vitamin C: 0mg

- Calcium: 6mg
- Iron: 0mg

CHOCOLATE- ICED MOCHA

Prep Time: 6 minutes
Serving Per: 1 servings
Ready In: 6 minutes
Calories: 105

Ingredients
☐ 1 14 cups cold coffee, divided

☐ 1 envelope low-calorie hot cocoa mix ice cubes, or as needed

☐ 12 cup unsweetened almond milk

☐ 2 tablespoons sugar-free chocolate syrup, or more to taste

Directions
Heat 14 cup coffee in microwave in a mug until warmed, about 30 seconds. Stir cocoa mix into the coffee until dissolved.

Fill a large glass with ice cubes. Pour 1 cup cold coffee and almond milk over the ice cubes; stir the cocoa mixture and chocolate syrup into the coffee and almond milk.

Nutrition Info
- Total Fat: 1.8g   3 %

- Saturated Fat: 0g
- Cholesterol: 3mg   < 1 %
- Sodium: 255mg   10 %
- Potassium: 532mg   15 %
- Total Carbohydrates: 16.7g   5 %
- Dietary Fiber: 1.3g   5 %
- Protein: 5.2g   10 %

BOWL OF OATMEAL COOKIE

"A spruced up version of a bowl of oatmeal that tastes more like an oatmeal cookie! I make mine in the microwave for a quick and easy breakfast."

Prep Time: 5 minutes
Cook: 3 minutes
Serving Per: 2 servings
Ready In: 8 minutes
Calories: 292

Ingredients

- [ ] <u>1 egg 1 cup milk</u>
- [ ] 3 tablespoons milk
- [ ] 23 cup quick-cooking oats
- [ ] 2 tablespoons raisins, or to taste (optional)
- [ ] 1 tablespoon brown sugar

- ☐ 1 teaspoon vanilla extract
- ☐ 1 teaspoon butter, or to taste
- ☐ 14 teaspoon ground cinnamon salt to taste

Directions

Beat egg in a microwave-safe bowl; add 1 cup plus 3 tablespoons milk, oats, raisins, brown sugar, vanilla extract, butter, cinnamon, and salt and mix well.

Microwave on high for 1 minute; stir and microwave for 1 minute more. Stir oatmeal and microwave until cooked, about 1 minute more.

Nutrition Info

- Total Fat: 9.2g   14 %
- Saturated Fat: 4.0g
- Cholesterol: 110mg   37 %
- Sodium: 114mg   5 %
- Potassium: 440mg   12 %
- Total Carbohydrates: 40.6g   13 %
- Dietary Fiber: 3.3g   13 %
- Protein: 11.8g   24 %

ASIAN NOODLE SALAD

"This is a beautiful and flavorful salad with a fresh ginger dressing. The cap of the shiitake mushroom has a meaty flesh with a lot of flavor; reserve the tough stems for stocks. White or cremini mushrooms can be substituted. These are less expensive but not as flavorful."

Prep Time: 15 minutes
Cook: 8 minutes
Serving Per: 4 servings
Ready In: 23 minutes
Calories: 230

Ingredients
- [ ] 8 ounces capellini pasta
- [ ] 12 pound shiitake mushrooms
- [ ] 1 red bell pepper, thinly sliced
- [ ] 14 cup rice vinegar
- [ ] 3 tablespoons soy sauce1 tablespoon vegetable oil
- [ ] 1 teaspoon grated fresh ginger
- [ ] 1 tablespoon chopped fresh parsley

Directions
Cook pasta in a large pot of boiling water. Meanwhile, clean, stem, and slice mushrooms. Add mushrooms and red bell pepper during last 2 minutes of cooking. Drain.

In a small bowl, mix together vinegar, soy sauce, oil, and ginger.

Transfer pasta, mushrooms, and pepper to a serving bowl; toss with ginger dressing. Sprinkle with parsley before serving.

Nutrition Info

- Total Fat: 4.8g   7 %
- Saturated Fat: 1.0g
- Cholesterol: 41mg   14 %
- Sodium: 705mg   28 %
- Potassium: 196mg   5 %
- Total Carbohydrates: 36.6g   12 %
- Dietary Fiber: 3.5g   14 %
- Protein: 8.7g   17 %
- Sugars: 2g
- Vitamin A: 1037IU
- Vitamin C: 41mg

WHOLEWHEAT SPAGHETTI WITH SARDINES AND CHERRY TOMATOES

Prep time: 10 minutes
Serving Per: 2 serves (generous portions)
Cooking time: 15 minutes
Calories: 502

Ingredients

- ☐ 150-175g (5 12 - 6oz) dried wholewheat spaghetti
- ☐ 2 teaspoons olive oil
- ☐ 1 small red onion, finely chopped
- ☐ 1 clove garlic, crushed (optional)
- ☐ A good pinch or two of dried chilli flakes

- ☐ 175g (6oz) ripe cherry tomatoes, halved
- ☐ 85g (3oz) frozen peas
- ☐ 150ml (14 pint) passata
- ☐ 120g (4 14oz) can sardines in tomato sauce
- ☐ 1 teaspoon shredded fresh basil leaves, plus extra to garnish
- ☐ Freshly ground black pepper, to taste

Directions

Cook spaghetti in a large pan of boiling water for 10-12 minutes or according to packet instructions, until tender.

Meanwhile, make sauce. Heat olive oil in a non-stick saucepan; add onion and garlic (if using) and sauté for 5-7 minutes or until onion is softened.

Stir in chilli flakes, tomatoes, peas, passata and sardines with their sauce, breaking up sardines roughly. Cover and simmer for about 5 minutes or until sauce is hot and tomatoes are softened. Stir in basil; season with black pepper.

Drain spaghetti, reserving 2 tablespoons of the cooking water; add reserved cooking water to sardine sauce in pan. Add spaghetti to sauce, toss to mix well. Serve immediately, sprinkled with extra shredded basil.

Cook's tips

Try dried white or spinach pasta (such as spaghetti, tagliatelle, fusilli or penne) instead of wholewheat spaghetti, or use another type of dried wholewheat pasta (such as as fusilli or penne).

Substitute sardines with canned mackerel fillets in tomato sauce.
Try using frozen (defrosted) baby broad beans or sweetcorn kernels in place of the peas. Serve with a dark green leaf salad if you like.

Nutrition Info

- Total Fat: 12.2g 17 %
- Saturated Fat: 2.7g   14 %
- Energy (kcal): 502   25 %
- Sugar: 11.2g   12 %
- Salt: 0.8g 13 %

CHAPTER THREE

SALMON PATE ON WHOLEGRAIN TOAST

Prep time: 10 minutes
Serving Per: 4 serves
Cooking time: None
Calories: 413

Ingredients

- [ ] 225g (8oz) cold poached (skinless) salmon fillet
- [ ] 6 teaspoons quark (or very low-fat soft cheese)
- [ ] 1 teaspoon creamed horseradish sauce (use a gluten-free brand if you like)
- [ ] 1 teaspoon finely grated lemon zest
- [ ] 1 teaspoon finely chopped fresh parsley
- [ ] 1 teaspoon finely snipped fresh chives
- [ ] Freshly ground black pepper, to taste
- [ ] Wholegrain bread or toast, to serve (use a gluten-free brand if you like). Watercress sprigs, to garnish

Directions

Flake salmon into a bowl. Add quark and mash together.
Add horseradish sauce, lemon zest, herbs and black pepper; mix well.
Serve with crusty bread or toast and garnish with watercress sprigs.

Dietary tips

Make it gluten-free by using gluten-free horseradish sauce and serving with gluten-free bread, crackers or vegetable crudites

Nutrition Info

- Total Fat: 6.8g   14 %
- Saturated Fat: 1.6g   8 %
- Energy (kcal): 413   21 %
- Sugar: 6.5g   7 %
- Salt: 1.5g   25 %

FLAVORED LATTE

"Use this basic recipe to make your favorite flavored latte with a home espresso machine."
Prep Time: 4 minutes
Cook : 1 minutes
Serving Per: 1 servings
Ready In: 5 minutes
Calories: 105

Ingredients

☐   1 14 cups 2% milk

☐   2 tablespoons any flavor of flavored syrup

☐   1 (1.5 fluid ounce) jigger brewed espresso

Directions

Pour milk into a steaming pitcher and heat to 145 degrees F to 165 degrees F (65 to 70 degrees C) using the steaming wand. Measure the flavored syrup into a large coffee mug. Brew espresso, then add to mug. Pour the steamed milk into the mug, using a spoon to hold back the foam. Spoon foam over the top.

Nutrition Info

- Total Fat: 6.1g   9 %
- Saturated Fat: 4.0g
- Cholesterol: 24mg   8 %
- Sodium: 142mg   6 %
- Potassium: 518mg   14 %
- Total Carbohydrates: 41.3g   13 %
- Dietary Fiber: 0g   0 %
- Protein: 10.1g   20 %
- Sugars: 33g
- Vitamin A: 576IU
- Vitamin C: 1mg
- Calcium: 360mg
- Iron: 0mg
- Thiamin: 0mg
- Niacin: 4mg
- Vitamin B6: 0mg
- Magnesium: 69mg
- Folate: 16mcg

OKRA CURRY (BHINDI OR BHINDA)

Prep time: 5-10 minutes
Serving Per: 6 serves
Cooking time: 10-20 minutes
Calories:65

Ingredients
- [ ] 450g 1lb okra
- [ ] 1 tablespoon olive oil
- [ ] 1 teaspoon cumin seeds
- [ ] 2 medium onions, chopped
- [ ] 1 teaspoon green chillies, crushed
- [ ] 1 1/2 teaspoons cumin coriander powder
- [ ] 1/2 teaspoon turmeric powder
- [ ] 1 medium tomato, chopped
- [ ] 1 tablespoon coriander leaves and stalks, chopped separately
- [ ] 1 tablespoon lemon juice (optional)

Cook's tips

When buying okra, look for small pods which is the most tender and ensure the skin is nice and fresh - not dry looking. If a pod snaps when bent, it is fresh.

Wash each okra under cold running water (there's no need to dry them). Cut them into pieces 1cm-2.5cm or 1/2-1in long. Set to one side.

In a large, non-stick pan, heat the oil, add the cumin seeds and chopped onions and cook until the onions are soft.

Add the okra, green chillies, cumin coriander powder, turmeric and chopped coriander stalks. Mix well.

Spoon the tomato on top of the okra mixture and cook uncovered for 5 minutes on a medium heat. Toss the okra every 2-3 minutes after this. Lower the heat and cook for 7-10 minutes or until cooked.

Remove from the heat and place in a serving dish. Garnish with the chopped coriander leaves and sprinkle the lemon juice over the dish just before serving.

Nutrition info

- Total Fat: 3.1g   1 %
- Saturated Fat: 0.2g   1 %
- Energy (kcal): 65   3 %
- Sugar: 4.5g   5 %
- Salt: 0.3g   1 %

AMAZING MEXICAN QUINOA SALAD

"Extremely yummy, spicy marinated salad that will keep in the fridge for up to a week! My kids in university love packing this up for their lunch. You have everything you need for a very healthy meal in one dish! Substitute barley for the brown rice if desired. Turtle beans can be substituted for kidney beans."

Prep Time: 20 minutes
Cook: 2 hours
Serving Per: 8 servings
Ready In: 2h 20 minutes
Calories: 397

Ingredients

- ☐ 2 cups cooked quinoa
- ☐ 1 (15 ounce) can pinto beans, rinsed and drained
- ☐ 1 (15 ounce) can kidney beans, rinsed and drained
- ☐ 1 (14 ounce) can corn1 red onion, chopped
- ☐ 1 cup cooked brown rice
- ☐ 1 red bell pepper, chopped
- ☐ 14 cup chopped fresh cilantroDressing:34 cup olive oil
- ☐ 13 cup red wine vinegar
- ☐ 1 tablespoon chili powder, or to taste
- ☐ 2 cloves garlic, mashed
- ☐ 12 teaspoon salt
- ☐ 12 teaspoon ground black pepper
- ☐ 14 teaspoon cayenne pepper, or to taste

Directions

Mix quinoa, pinto beans, kidney beans, corn, red onion, brown rice, red bell pepper, and cilantro together in a glass or plastic container with a lid.

Whisk olive oil, vinegar, chili powder, garlic, salt, black pepper, and cayenne pepper together in a bowl; pour over quinoa mixture and toss to coat. Cover bowl with a lid and refrigerate until flavors blend, at least 2 hours. Stir again before serving.

Nutrition Info

- Total Fat: 22.6g   35 %
- Saturated Fat: 3.0g
- Cholesterol: 0mg   0 %
- Sodium: 532mg   21 %
- Potassium: 272mg   8 %
- Total Carbohydrates: 42.4g   14 %
- Dietary Fiber: 8.6g   34 %
- Protein: 9.1g   18 %

LUNCHBOX FRIENDLY NUT-FREE COOKIES
Prep time: 25 minutes
Serving Per: 12 serves
Cooking time: 10 minutes
Ready in: 35 minutes

Ingredients
- ☐   <u>2 smashed ripe bananas</u>
- ☐   1 teaspoon vanilla extract
- ☐   1 teaspoon ground cinnamon
- ☐   60 ml extra virgin olive oil or coconut oil
- ☐   60 ml organic maple syrup
- ☐   150 g rolled organic oats
- ☐   100 g desiccated coconut
- ☐   100 g sultanas
- ☐   1 apple, finely chopped

- ☐ 14 cup Healthy Chef Protein (you can use Natural or Vanilla in these cookies)
- ☐ Generous pinch sea salt

Directions

PREHEAT your oven to 160°C 320°F – fan-forced.
COMBINE smashed banana, vanilla, cinnamon, olive oil and maple syrup.
ADD oats, coconut, sultanas, apples, Healthy Chef Protein and sea salt.
Mix together well and allow to sit for 5 minutes to allow the oats to soften.
FORM into 12 cookies. I like to use a small ice-cream scoop for this.
BAKE for 30 – 35 minutes or until golden.
COOL and enjoy.

CHAPTER FOUR

Warm Wild Berry Buckle from the Berry Basket

Prep time: 25 minutes
Serving Per: 8 serves
Cooking time: 10 minutes
Ready in: 35 minutes

Ingredients

- [ ] <u>Berry Compote</u>
- [ ] 2 tablespoons lemon juice
- [ ] 3 tablespoons orange juice
- [ ] 12 cup sugar
- [ ] 2 tablespoons cornstarch
- [ ] 12 cup frozen blackberries, thawed
- [ ] 12 cup frozen raspberries, thawed
- [ ] 12 cup frozen blueberries, thawed
- [ ] 2 cups quartered fresh strawberries, divided
- [ ] 2 cups fresh blueberries

Oatmeal Streusel Ingredients

- [ ] <u>13 cup all-purpose flour</u>
- [ ] 1 tablespoon ground cinnamon
- [ ] 14 cup brown sugar
- [ ] 13 cup oatmeal

- [ ] 12 cup butter, melted

Directions
1. Combine lemon juice, orange juice, sugar, and cornstarch in a large bowl.
Add thawed blackberries, raspberries, blueberries, and 1 cup of the fresh strawberries. Puree using an immersion blender until smooth.
2. Gently fold in the fresh blueberries and remaining 1 cup of strawberries.
3. Set aside.

Baking Instructions
1. Place 13 cup of cake batter in the bottom of each prepared ramekin.
2. Top with 13 cup of berry compote.
3. Bake for 25-30 minutes, until cake is set.

PARCHMENT BAKED SALMON

Prep time: 15 minutes
Serving Per: 2 serves
Cooking time: 25 minutes
Ready in: 40 minutes
"Salmon baked in parchment paper is the best way to steam in great taste."

Ingredients
- [ ] 1 (8 ounce) salmon filled salt and ground black pepper to taste
- [ ] 14 cup chopped basil leavesolive oil cooking spray
- [ ] 1 lemon, thinly sliced

☐ Add all ingredients to list

Directions

Place an oven rack in the lowest position in oven and preheat oven to 400 degrees F (200 degrees C).

Place salmon fillet with skin side down in the middle of a large piece of parchment paper; season with salt and black pepper. Cut 2 3-inch slits into the fish with a sharp knife. Stuff chopped basil leaves into the slits. Spray fillet with cooking spray and arrange lemon slices on top.

Fold edges of parchment paper over the fish several times to seal into an airtight packet. Place sealed packet onto a baking sheet.

Bake fish on the bottom rack of oven until salmon flakes easily and meat is pink and opaque with an interior of slightly darker pink color, about 25 minutes. An instant-read meat thermometer inserted into the thickest part of

the fillet should read at least 145 degrees F (65 degrees C). To serve, cut the parchment paper open and remove lemon slices before plating fish.

Nutrition Info

- Total Fat: 6.9g   11 %
- Saturated Fat: 1.0g
- Cholesterol: 50mg   17 %
- Sodium: 48mg   2 %
- Potassium: 495mg   14 %
- Total Carbohydrates: 6.1g   2 %
- Dietary Fiber: 2.7g   11 %

- Protein: 24.8g   50 %

GINGER GLAZED MAHI MAHI

"This Ginger Glazed Mahi Mahi is bursting with flavor and combines both sweet and sour taste sensations. The 30 minute prep time includes 20 minutes to marinate. This recipe is a snap and so delicious. You'll love it!"

Prep time: 5 minutes
Serving Per: 4 serves
Cooking time: 12 minutes
Ready in: 37 minutes
Calories: 259

Ingredients

☐   3 tablespoons honey

☐   3 tablespoons soy sauce

☐   3 tablespoons balsamic vinegar

☐   1 teaspoon grated fresh ginger root

☐   1 clove garlic, crushed or to taste

☐   2 teaspoons olive oil

☐   4 (6 ounce) mahi mahi fillets salt and pepper to taste

☐   1 tablespoon vegetable oil

Directions

In a shallow glass dish, stir together the honey, soy sauce, balsamic vinegar, ginger, garlic and olive oil. Season fish fillets with salt and pepper, and place them into the dish. If the fillets have skin on them, place them skin side down.

Cover, and refrigerate for 20 minutes to marinate.

Heat vegetable oil in a large skillet over medium-high heat. Remove fish from the dish, and reserve marinade. Fry fish for 4 to 6 minutes on each side, turning only once, until fish flakes easily with a fork. Remove fillets to a serving platter and keep warm.

Pour reserved marinade into the skillet, and heat over medium heat until the mixture reduces to a glaze consistently. Spoon glaze over fish, and serve immediately.

Nutrition Info

- Total Fat: 7g 11 %
- Saturated Fat: 1.0g
- Cholesterol: 124mg 41 %
- Sodium: 830mg 33 %
- Potassium: 755mg 21 %
- Total Carbohydrates: 16g   5 %
- Dietary Fiber: 0.2g   < 1 %
- Protein: 32.4g   65 %

P ESTO CHICKEN FLORENTINE

"Extremely rich combination of chicken, spinach and creamy pesto sauce. Serve with crunchy bread and romaine salad--it's the best!"

Prep time: 20 minutes
Serving Per: 4 serves
Cooking time: 35 minutes
Ready in: 55 minutes
Calories: 572

Ingredients

- [ ] 2 tablespoons olive oil
- [ ] 2 cloves garlic, finely chopped
- [ ] 4 skinless, boneless chicken breast halves - cut into strips
- [ ] 2 cups fresh spinach leaves1 (4.5 ounce)
- [ ] package dry Alfredo sauce mix
- [ ] 2 tablespoons pesto
- [ ] 1 (8 ounce) package dry penne pasta
- [ ] 1 tablespoon grated Romano cheese

Directions

Heat oil in a large skillet over medium high heat. Add garlic, saute for 1 minute; then add chicken and cook for 7 to 8 minutes on each side. When chicken is close to being cooked through (no longer pink inside), add spinach and saute all together for 3 to 4 minutes.

Meanwhile, prepare Alfredo sauce according to package directions. When finished, stir in 2 tablespoons pesto; set aside.

In a large pot of salted boiling water, cook pasta for 8 to 10 minutes or until aldente. Rinse under cold water and drain.

Add chickenspinach mixture to pasta, then stir in pestoAlfredo sauce.

Mix well, top with cheese and serve.

Nutrition Info

- Total Fat: 19.3g 30 %
- Saturated Fat: 6.0g
- Cholesterol: 84mg 28 %
- Sodium: 1707mg 68 %
- Potassium: 520mg 15 %
- Total Carbohydrates: 57.3g   18 %
- Dietary Fiber: 2.5g   10 %
- Protein: 41.9g   84 %

BLACK BEANS AND RICE

Prep time: 5 minutes
Serving Per: 10 serves
Cooking time: 25 minutes
Ready in: 30 minutes
Calories: 140

Ingredients

- ☐ 1 teaspoon olive oil1 onion, chopped
- ☐ 2 cloves garlic, minced
- ☐ 34 cup uncooked white rice
- ☐ 1 12 cups low sodium, low fat vegetable broth
- ☐ 1 teaspoon ground cumin
- ☐ 14 teaspoon cayenne pepper
- ☐ 3 12 cups canned black beans, drained

Directions

In a stockpot over medium-high heat, heat the oil. Add the onion and garlic and saute for 4 minutes. Add the rice and saute for 2 minutes.
Add the vegetable broth, bring to a boil, cover and lower the heat and cook for 20 minutes. Add the spices and black beans.

Nutrition Info

- Total Fat: 0.9g 1 %
- Saturated Fat: 0.0g
- Cholesterol: 0mg 0 %
- Sodium: 354mg 14 %
- Potassium: 298mg 8 %
- Total Carbohydrates: 27.1g   9 %
- Dietary Fiber: 6.2g   25 %
- Protein: 6.3g 13 %

CONCLUSION

There is a ton of information out there but trying to zero in on the best healthy meal recipes for you and your family is going to take time. You also have to be prepared to make a lot of changes until you find something that works for everyone. I used to joke about our kids' reaction to some of my dishes (Ginger Glazed Mahi Mahi soup comes to mind) - if they don't like it, it must be good for you!

Seriously though, there are lots of good healthy dinner recipes available that everyone will love. You just need to be able to spend the time to find them, and experiment a little in the kitchen.

www.ingramcontent.com/pod-product-compliance
Lightning Source LLC
Chambersburg PA
CBHW071445070526
44578CB00001B/211